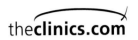

HEART FAILURE CLINICS

The Role of Surgery, Part II

GUEST EDITORS
Stephen Westaby, MS, PhD
Mario C. Deng, MD

CONSULTING EDITORS
Jagat Narula, MD, PhD
James B. Young, MD

July 2007 • Volume 3 • Number 3

SAUNDERS

An Imprint of Elsevier, Inc.
PHILADELPHIA   LONDON   TORONTO   MONTREAL   SYDNEY   TOKYO

W.B. SAUNDERS COMPANY
A Division of Elsevier Inc.

1600 John F. Kennedy Boulevard. • Suite 1800 • Philadelphia, Pennsylvania 19103-2899

http://www.theclinics.com

HEART FAILURE CLINICS
July 2007
Editor: Barbara Cohen-Kligerman

Volume 3, Number 3
ISSN 1551-7136
ISBN-13: 978-1-4160-5477-1
ISBN-10: 1-4160-5477-4

Reprints: For copies of 100 or more, or articles in this publication, please contact the Commercial Reprints Department, Elsevier Inc., 360 Park Avenue South, New York, New York 10010-1710. Tel.: (+1) 212-633-3813; Fax: (+1) 212-462-1935; e-mail: reprints@elsevier.com.

The ideas and opinions expressed in *Heart Failure Clinics* do not necessarily reflect those of the Publisher. The Publisher does not assume any responsibility for any injury and/or damage to persons or property arising out of or related to any use of the material contained in this periodical. The reader is advised to check the appropriate medical literature and the product information currently provided by the manufacturer of each drug to be administered to verify the dosage, the method and duration of administration, or contraindications. It is the responsibility of the treating physician or other health care professional, relying on independent experience and knowledge of the patient, to determine drug dosages and the best treatment for the patient. Mention of any product in this issue should not be construed as endorsement by the contributors, editors, or the Publisher of the product or manufacturers' claims.

Heart Failure Clinics (ISSN 1551-7136) is published quarterly by Elsevier Inc., 360 Park Avenue South, New York, NY 10010-1710. Months of publication are January, April, July, and October. Business and editorial offices: 1600 John F. Kennedy Boulevard, Suite 1800, Philadelphia, PA 19103-2899. Customer service office: 6277 Sea Harbor Drive, Orlando, FL 32887-4800. Periodicals postage paid at New York, NY and additional mailing offices. Subscription prices are USD 157 per year for US individuals, USD 260 per year for US institutions, USD 54 per year for US students and residents, USD 189 per year for Canadian individuals, USD 292 per year for Canadian institutions, USD 189 per year for international individuals, USD 292 per year for international institutions and USD 65 per year for foreign students/residents. To receive student and resident rate, orders must be accompanied by name of affiliated institution, date of term, and the *signature* of program/residency coordinator on institution letterhead. Orders will be billed at individual rate until proof of status is received. Foreign air speed delivery is included in all *Clinics* subscription prices. All prices are subject to change without notice. POSTMASTER: Send address changes to *Heart Failure Clinics*, Elsevier Periodicals Customer Service, 6277 Sea Harbor Drive, Orlando, FL 32887-4800. **Customer Service: 1-800-654-2452 (US). From outside of the US, call (+1) 407-345-4000.**

Heart Failure Clinics is covered in *Index Medicus*.

Printed in the United States of America.

Cover artwork courtesy of Umberto M. Jezek.

CONSULTING EDITORS

JAGAT NARULA, MD, PhD, Professor, Medicine; Chief, Division of Cardiology; and Associate Dean, University of California Irvine School of Medicine, Orange, California

JAMES B. YOUNG, MD, Chairman and Professor, Department of Medicine, Lerner College of Medicine; and George and Linda Kaufman Chair, Cleveland Clinic Foundation, Case Western Reserve University, Cleveland, Ohio

INCOMING CONSULTING EDITOR

RAGAVENDRA R. BALIGA, MD, MBA, FRCP, FACC, Director, Section of Cardiovascular Medicine, University Hospital East; and Clinical Professor, Internal Medicine, The Ohio State University, Columbus, Ohio

GUEST EDITORS

STEPHEN WESTABY, MS, PhD, FRCS, Professor, Oxford Heart Centre, John Radcliffe Hospital, Headington, Oxford, United Kingdom

MARIO C. DENG, MD, FACC, FESC, Center for Advanced Cardiac Care, College of Physicians and Surgeons, Columbia University, New York, New York

CONTRIBUTORS

STEVEN F. BOLLING, MD, Section of Cardiac Surgery, University of Michigan, Ann Arbor, Michigan

MARTIN CADEIRAS, MD, College of Physicians and Surgeons, Columbia University, New York, New York

ANDREW L. CLARK, MD, University of Hull, Castle Hill Hospital, Kingston-upon-Hull, United Kingdom

JOHN CLELAND, MD, FESC, FACC, University of Hull, Castle Hill Hospital, Kingston-upon-Hull, United Kingdom

REYNOLDS M. DELGADO III, MD, Mechanical Assist Devices in Heart Failure, The Texas Heart Institute at St. Luke's Episcopal Hospital, Houston, Texas

MARIO C. DENG, MD, FACC, FESC, Center for Advanced Cardiac Care, College of Physicians and Surgeons, Columbia University, New York, New York

NEIL HOBSON, MBBS, University of Hull, Castle Hill Hospital, Kingston-upon-Hull, United Kingdom

OLGA KHALEVA, MD, Department of Cardiology, University of Hull, Castle Hill Hospital, Kingston-upon-Hull, United Kingdom

JOHANNES MUELLER, MD, Dip.-Ing. (TU), Berlin Heart, Berlin, Germany

PHILIP A. POOLE-WILSON, MD, FRCP, FMedSci, British Heart Foundation Simon Marks Professor of Cardiology, Cardiac Medicine, National Heart & Lung Institute, Imperial College London, London, United Kingdom

MANUEL PRINZ von BAYERN, PhD, College of Physicians and Surgeons, Columbia University, New York, New York

BRANISLAV RADOVANCEVIC, MD, Center for Cardiac Support; and Associate Director, Cardiovascular Surgery and Transplant Research, The Texas Heart Institute at St. Luke's Episcopal Hospital, Houston, Texas

HARRY RAKOWSKI, MD, FRCPC, FACC, E. Douglas Wigle Chair in Hpertrophic Cardiomyopathy and Professor of Medicine, Division of Cardiology, University of Toronto, Toronto General Hospital, Toronto, Ontario, Canada

†MARTINUS T. SPOOR, MD, formerly of the Section of Cardiac Surgery, University of Michigan, Ann Arbor, Michigan

AHMED TAGELDIEN, MSc, MD, University of Hull, Castle Hill Hospital, Kingston-upon-Hull, United Kingdom

GERD WALLUKAT, PhD, Max Delbrueck Center, Berlin, Germany

STEPHEN WESTABY, MS, PhD, FRCS, Professor, Oxford Heart Centre, John Radcliffe Hospital, Headington, Oxford, United Kingdom

ANNA WOO, MD, SM, FRCPC, FACC, Assistant Professor of Medicine, Division of Cardiology, University of Toronto, Toronto General Hospital, Toronto, Ontario, Canada

---

† Deceased.

CONTENTS

In patients who have end-stage heart failure, medical therapy is of limited use, and heart transplantation is frequently not an option because of the shortage of donor hearts. Two new treatment options, left ventricular assist devices (LVADs) and implantable cardiac resynchronization therapy (CRT) devices, can improve survival and quality of life in patients who have heart failure. Both types of devices are easy to implant. However, LVADs carry the risk of infection and mechanical failure, and CRT is ineffective in a substantial proportion of patients who have heart failure. Therefore, methods must be devised to identify patients who have heart failure who are likely to benefit from these devices. Data suggest that early LVAD implantation, before end-stage heart failure develops, is critical to slowing or reversing disease progression. Similarly, in indicated patients who have less advanced disease, CRT may be particularly beneficial.

Currently, cardiac resynchronization therapy (CRT) should be considered before a left ventricular assist device for most patients who have moderate or severe left ventricular systolic dysfunction and have not responded symptomatically to conventional pharmacologic measures. There is little evidence that the severity of cardiac dyssynchrony as measured using current techniques is useful in predicting the benefits of CRT. QRS duration on the surface ECG is a surrogate marker of the severity of the left ventricular ejection fraction as well as of several types of dyssynchrony. More clinical trials are required to determine whether excluding patients who have QRS duration less than 120 msec or those who have no evidence of dyssynchrony from implantation of CRT is appropriate. Perhaps all patients who have moderate or severe left ventricular systolic dysfunction should be considered for CRT, either to improve symptoms if they are persistent or relapsing, or to improve outcome. In the longer-term future, it is possible that the development of less expensive, small, and safe left ventricular assist devices will supplant the role of both CRT and CRT-defibrillator devices.

FORTHCOMING ISSUES

RECENT ISSUES

Heart Failure Clin 3 (2007) ix–x

Editorial

A Beloved Daughter at Two and a Half

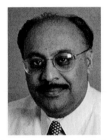

Jagat Narula, MD, PhD
Consulting Editor

We know what a sweet little daughter means to a doting Daddy. We know how a Daddy feels when he walks with his little lady, steadfastly holding that little finger on her soft, tiny hand. We know how his heart warms up when he beholds his baby daughter running excitedly up to him, clutching his knees, clamoring to be gathered up in his arms, and hugged and kissed. We know how happy he gets as he stokes her hair and lulls her to sleep, the little lady perched on his knees, her head and cheek nestled on his chest.

We have raised the *Heart Failure Clinics* (HFC) with similar affection. HFC was the first in the latest generation of *Clinics*, born two and a half years ago. The *Clinics of North America* were initiated 95 years ago with the objective of consolidating established and current literature about a selected disease entity to provide diagnostic and management guidelines for practicing physicians and trainees. The popularity of the *Clinics* series has led to subspecialty *Clinics,* such as *Cardiology Clinics,* and, subsequently, to the third generation of *Clinics,* such as HFC.

Since April 2005, we have published quarterly HFC issues ranging from purely clinical to essentially translational and basic science topics. We have invited 15 guest editors and more than 200 authors, who have brought you the highest level and most sophisticated subject information. We are grateful to our guest editors and contributors

for their efforts. We tried to start the series with relatively broad topics, such as neurohumoral antagonists in the management of heart failure, cardiovascular imaging techniques, myocarditis, and the pathogenesis of heart failure. Our plan is to gradually turn to more focused topics such as statins in heart failure, use of stem cell therapy, and myocardial architecture. We hope that you have enjoyed the attractive appearance of HFC. Audience surveys indicate that you have appreciated our unorthodox editorials, discussing one or two specific controversies related to the theme of that particular issue and highlighting manuscripts that we hope stimulated readers to think outside of the box. We have worked hard to ensure that article contents were not repetitive, which was particularly difficult because all articles revolved around a single theme. We are particularly proud of the fact that HFC was accepted by the National Library of Medicine for citation in PubMed in a very short time, and that its readership has grown tremendously.

This is the last issue of HFC for which I am serving as the Consulting Editor. I have thoroughly enjoyed seeing it grow. I will start as the Editor-in-Chief of the *Journal of the American College of Cardiology: Cardiovascular Imaging* beginning July 1, 2007. I would like to offer my sincere gratitude to my co-editor, Jim Young, with whom I have enjoyed working and have

doi:10.1016/j.hfc.2007.07.001

heartfailure.theclinics.com

developed a close bond of friendship. I will particularly miss his Blackberry e-mail notes, which
waited for me every morning when I woke up.
He fully took advantage of the 3-hour time difference between Cleveland and California. I am also
thankful to my executive editors, initially Heather
Cullen and then Karen Sorenson, who have
worked with me tirelessly and never complained
about my calls at odd hours. While Jim took advantage of the Eastern Time zone, Karen and
Heather suffered because they were awakened at
night when I settled to work on HFC every even-
ing in California.

Jim will have a very capable co-editor in
Ragavendra Baliga from Ohio State University.

And, fortunately, HFC will not be split between
parents from across the country anymore. Barbara Cohen-Kligerman, another very experienced
executive editor, will carry on with Karen's
position. Although I know that I will miss my
day-to-day interaction with HFC, I am happy
that it is in very able hands. As I watch the toddler
grow to maturity, I know it will be a source of
pleasure to you all as it has been to me.

Jagat Narula, MD, PhD
University of California
Irvine, CA, USA

E-mail address: Narula@uci.edu

ELSEVIER
SAUNDERS

Heart Failure Clin 3 (2007) xi–xii

HEART
FAILURE
CLINICS

Editorial

Evolution Is Longer Lasting Than Revolution: Onward With *Heart Failure Clinics*

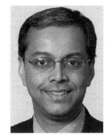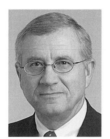

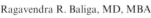

Ragavendra R. Baliga, MD, MBA   James B. Young, MD
Consulting Editors

Because of the devastating impact that heart failure has on patients from a morbidity, mortality, and economic standpoint, getting the message out about how best to understand, prevent, and treat the condition is essential. Indeed, heart failure affects approximately 5 million Americans and is the only major cardiovascular disorder on the rise. About 500,000 new cases of heart failure are diagnosed each year, and the number of deaths in the United States from this condition has more than doubled since 1979, averaging 250,000 annually. Less than 50% of patients are alive at 5 years after their initial diagnosis of congestive heart failure, and less than 25% are alive at 10 years.

Recognizing the need for increasing awareness about heart failure, *Heart Failure Clinics* was established two and half years ago, with Dr. Jagat Narula and Dr. James B. Young as the founding Consulting Editors. Very rapidly, it has met its expectation of being a "go-to" publication for community physicians and clinicians-in-training who are interested in a concise overview of topics related to heart failure. Its widespread acceptance

and readership resulted in it being listed in *Index Medicus* in the record time of 2 years.

The bulk of the credit for early success goes to Jagat Narula, who is widely recognized for his extraordinary energy, intellect, and wisdom. He was not only able to leverage his personal relationships with leaders in heart failure, such as William Dec and Gregg Fonarow, but also with those in other interdisciplinary fields, such as Blase Carabello, Roger Hajjar, Vasken Dilsizian, Mario Garcia, Stephen Westaby, John Burnett, and many others, to cover areas that were critical to understanding the nuances of heart failure diagnosis, treatment, and prevention. These efforts have resulted in *Heart Failure Clinics* now being positioned at the front of line of publications for those professionals whose lives involve treating and managing heart failure.

Despite its early success, *Heart Failure Clinics* continues to face challenges and opportunities in this ever-changing world of transmission of content and information. We recognize that, with time, knowledge will increasingly be delivered on-line, and *Heart Failure Clinics* already has an

1551-7136/07/$ - see front matter © 2007 Elsevier Inc. All rights reserved.
doi:10.1016/j.hfc.2007.07.002

heartfailure.theclinics.com

electronic version of its contents. As *Heart Failure Clinics* continues to grow, we plan to increase functionality of its website.

Also, there has been a changing of the guard, with Jagat becoming an emeritus editor in view of his new position as Editor-in-Chief of the *Journal of the American College of Cardiology: Cardiovascular Imaging*. Furthermore, we now have Barbara Cohen-Kligerman as the new executive editor. Barbara is a veteran *Clinics* editor. Her experience and enthusiasm, and the fact that she has already hit the ground running, mean that *Heart Failure Clinics* should continue to flourish. We would also like to thank the previous executive editor, Karen Sorensen, for ensuring a smooth transition.

We wish Jagat continued success in his new role. Our goal for *Heart Failure Clinics* remains the same—to continue to provide cogent perspectives that will open up the field of heart failure to the front-line practicing clinician.

Ragavendra R. Baliga, MD, MBA, FRCP, FACC
Ohio State University
Columbus, Ohio, USA

E-mail address: Ragavendra.Baliga@osumc.edu

James B. Young, MD
Cleveland Clinic Foundation
Cleveland, Ohio, USA

E-mail address: youngj@ccf.org

ELSEVIER
SAUNDERS

Heart Failure Clin 3 (2007) xiii–xv

HEART
FAILURE
CLINICS

Preface

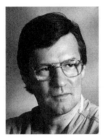   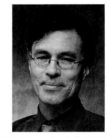

Stephen Westaby, MS, PhD, FRCS   Mario C. Deng, MD, FACC, FESC

Guest Editors

Worldwide, the heart failure syndrome has been increasing over the past decades, mainly because of the improved survival in acute heart attack situations in industrialized societies, as well as the epidemiologic transition in major parts of the world. The prevalence of heart failures is estimated to be around 1%–3% of the population. The advanced heart failure fraction of this group is estimated at 10%. In the United States of America and Europe alone, out of each population of greater than 300 million inhabitants, 3 to 5 million people who have heart failure and 300,000 to 500,000 people who have advanced heart failure have to face a situation with reduced survival probability as well as impaired quality of life and a functional status that is worse than the average prognosis of cancer.

Over the last three decades, based on an increasingly sophisticated understanding of the pathophysiology of the heart failure syndrome, therapeutic interventions have been tested in randomized clinical trials and implemented into clinical practice. Foremost, these have included the concept of neurohormonal blockade, which inhibits the chronic activation of the adrenergic nervous system by way of beta blockade, as well as inhibits the chronic activation of the renin-angiotensin-aldosterone system by angiotensin converting enzyme inhibitors, aldosterone receptor blockers, and aldosterone antagonists. Furthermore, interventional concepts, including defibrillator therapy and resynchronization pacemaker therapy, have been, after having shown the survival and quality of life benefit, implemented in clinical practice.

With respect to surgical treatment options in advanced heart failure, the situation in terms of evidence-based medicine has been less clear. For example, although heart transplantation—based on the initial spectacular success by Norman Shumway and colleagues at Stanford University—has been implemented in 300 centers around the world, it was never tested in a randomized clinical trial. More recently, the role of mechanical circulatory support therapy has been shown to yield a survival and quality of life benefit in advanced heart failure patients who are ineligible for heart transplantation. However, all other surgical options, including coronary artery bypass surgery, valvular surgery, and left ventricular volume reduction surgery, are based on observational series. In this situation, we would like to contribute, with this issue, an update of the status of surgical therapy in heart failure in order to reflect the best current

1551-7136/07/$ - see front matter © 2007 Elsevier Inc. All rights reserved.
doi:10.1016/j.hfc.2007.07.003

clinical practice patterns and clinical research directions. This issue comprises of a variety of articles that are provided by recognized authorities in their respective fields. Because of its overall volume, the issue is divided into Part I and Part II.

In the opening section of the first article, Sara Shumway reflects on the lifetime achievement of her father, Norman Shumway, who spearheaded the era of cardiac transplantation in the 1950s and 1960s, and has been a role model in terms of clinical practice, translated from basic and clinical research. In the second article, Howard Frazier pays tribute to Michael DeBakey a pioneer in cardiac surgery who, while alive and at the age of almost 100 years old, has been considered a living icon for everyone involved in the field of cardiac surgery by pioneering cardiac surgical techniques and technology, and by developing heart mechanical support, heart biological replacement, and the classification of aortic dissecting aneurysms. With respect to the diagnostic imaging approach to the heart failure patient in preparation of cardiac surgery, the article by Martin St. John Sutton provides an expert evaluation of imaging techniques that allow for definition of interventional strategies and risk evaluation. In his articles, Stephen Westaby provides a provocative insight into the question of whether today's cardiac surgery is a therapy for all heart failure patients, and outlines strategies to maximize the benefit of high-risk cardiac surgery in heart failure patients.

In the section on anti-ischemic surgical treatment options in heart failure, George Comas, Barry Esrig and Mehmet C. Oz provide an insight of the best practice patterns in patients who have acute coronary syndromes and life-threatening cardiogenic shock situations by surgical revascularization options. In the articles by Sorin V. Pusca and John D. Puscas, and by Ajay J. Kirtane and Jeffrey W. Moses, the debate on the topic of whether the cardiology interventional approaches with stent implantation or the cardiac surgical approach with coronary artery bypass grafting should be preferred is discussed. In their article, Lorenzo Menicanti and Marisa Di Donato outline the research scenario associated with the STICH trial that is attempting to answer the question of whether a revascularization approach with or without left ventricular volume restoration in heart failure patients is superior to current best management practice. Concluding this section is the article by William Sherman and colleagues, which outlines rationales that are underway in order to improve anti-ischemic

treatment by stem cell transplantation at the time of surgical or cardiology interventional maneuvers.

In the third section of the issue, on anti-arrhythmic and anti-pump failure interventions, Reynolds Delgado III advocates the LVAD approach for complete anti-arrhythmic treatment, while in their article, John Cleland, Ahmed Tageldien, Olga Khaleva, Neil Hobson, and Andrew L Clark argue for resynchronization therapy as a staged approach that has to precede more aggressive interventions. With respect to surgical treatment of hypertrophic cardiomyopathy, Anna Woo and Harry Rakowski summarize the experience utilizing myomectomy. In the final article of this section, Martinus Spoor[1] and Steven Bolling explain the rationales and analyze outcomes in patients who have advanced heart failure and are undergoing valve repair and replacement.

In the fourth section of the issue, in patients who have very advanced heart failure, beyond organ-saving anti-ischemic, anti–pump-failure, and anti-arrhythmic approaches, more complete heart replacement options are discussed. Johannes Mueller argues in favor of a weaning attempt for recovery in every patient who has undergone mechanical circulatory support implantation, while Philip A. Poole-Wilson makes a point that the low rate of recovery does not justify this weaning protocol in every situation. For patients who are potential candidates for heart transplantation, Martin Cadeiras, Manuel von Bayern, and Mario C. Deng critically review the potential benefit of heart transplantation in the context of contemporary alternatives in contrast to the situation 30 years ago when heart transplantation was developed, and the challenges to improve long-term mechanical circulatory support outcomes by improving the technology associated with pump development. The final article, by Stephen Westaby, argues the pros and cons of expansion of destination mechanical circulatory support centers beyond the current transplant centers.

We hope—based on this comprehensive review of the current expertise in surgical therapies for advanced heart failure in the framework of the specific decision-making algorithm that we as a team are facing with our patients everyday—that

---

[1] Martin Spoor, MD, died tragically in a plane crash on June 5, 2007 while retrieving a donor organ for heart transplantation.

this issue contributes to improvement in the field. We welcome your critical feedback.

Stephen Westaby, MS, PhD, FRCS
Oxford Heart Centre
John Radcliffe Hospital
Headley Way
Headington, Oxford OX3 9DU, UK

E-mail address: Stephen.westaby@orh.nhs.uk

Mario C. Deng, MD, FACC, FESC
Cardiac Transplantation Research
Department of Medicine
Division of Cardiology
Columbia University
622 West 168th Street
PH12 STEM, Room 134
New York, NY 10032, USA

E-mail address: md785@columbia.edu

ELSEVIER
SAUNDERS

Heart Failure Clin 3 (2007) 259–265

HEART
FAILURE
CLINICS

Symptomatic Relief: Left Ventricular Assist Devices Versus Resynchronization Therapy

Reynolds M. Delgado III, MD*, Branislav Radovancevic, MD

The Texas Heart Institute at St. Luke's Episcopal Hospital, Houston, Texas

The incidence of heart failure (HF) continues to grow because of the increasing number of elderly people and myocardial infarction survivors [1]. HF affects 4.7 million Americans and contributes to more than 250,000 deaths each year. More than 900,000 hospitalizations in 2002 were attributed to HF, and estimates of the annual cost of this disorder range from $10 billion to $40 billion [2].

Medical therapy is of limited use in patients who have HF. The investigators for the multicenter Randomized Evaluation of Mechanical Assistance for the Treatment of Congestive Heart Failure (REMATCH) trial found that mortality was 75% in patients receiving only medical therapy [3]. Although heart transplantation can help patients who have HF, its use is seriously constrained by the shortage of donor hearts. However, in addition to several drug treatments available for chronic HF, nonpharmacologic treatment, including device therapy, has become an effective and well-established treatment strategy for patients who have HF [1–3].

In addition to promoting survival, efforts to develop cardiac support devices have been aimed at improving the quality of life (QOL) of patients who have end-stage HF. Heart failure is associated with poor QOL because many of its symptoms, such as fatigue and shortness of breath, severely reduce patients' ability to perform their normal work, social, and leisure activities. Anxiety and depression are frequent and have a profound effect on patients' mental as well as physical health. These effects on patients' physical, cognitive, and emotional functioning may explain why ratings of physical and emotional QOL closely relate to their New York Heart Association (NYHA) classifications [4]. Because of this association, in the Heart Failure Society of America 2006 Comprehensive Heart Failure Guideline, improving symptoms and QOL is listed among the clinician's top priorities, along with slowing the progression of cardiac and peripheral dysfunction and reducing mortality, when treating patients who have HF and left ventricular systolic dysfunction.

Use of implanted devices is growing rapidly as a treatment option. Identifying patients who will benefit from device implantation and selecting the device that will be most advantageous for each patient is becoming more and more critical. Use of US Food and Drug Administration–approved devices in HF includes cardiac resynchronization therapy (CRT) and surgical implantation of mechanical circulatory assist devices. However, HF patient populations treated with these devices differ in their severity of illness, population size, and treatment options.

The left ventricular assist device (LVAD) is indicated for use as a bridge to transplantation in cardiac transplant candidates at risk of imminent death from irreversible left ventricular failure. The HeartMate XVE vented electric left ventricular assist system (LVAS) (Thoratec Corp., Pleasanton, California), which can be used inside and outside the hospital, is also indicated as a destination therapy for use in patients who have NYHA

* Corresponding author. The Texas Heart Institute at St. Luke's Episcopal Hospital, P.O. Box 20345, MC 2-114, Houston, TX 77225-0345.

E-mail address: rdelgado@heart.thi.tmc.edu (R.M. Delgado).

1551-7136/07/$ - see front matter © 2007 Elsevier Inc. All rights reserved.
doi:10.1016/j.hfc.2007.05.004

class IV end-stage left ventricular failure who are not candidates for cardiac transplantation and who have received optimal medical therapy for at least 60 of the last 90 days. To receive this LVAS, patients must also have a life expectancy of less than 2 years, a left ventricular ejection fraction (LVEF) of 25% or less, and a peak oxygen consumption of no more than 12 mL/kg/min or a continued need for intravenous inotropic therapy owing to symptomatic hypotension, decreasing renal function, or worsening pulmonary congestion. Likewise, CRT by biventricular pacing is indicated in selected patients who have NYHA functional class III or IV HF caused by idiopathic dilated or ischemic cardiomyopathy who have QRS duration 120 milliseconds or greater, left ventricular end-diastolic diameter 5.5 cm or greater, and ejection fraction 35% or less.

Symptom relief with a left ventricular assist device

The REMATCH trial showed the efficacy and safety of long-term LVAD support in patients who had chronic end-stage HF [3]. In terminally ill patients, LVAD recipients had better survival rates than did patients who received only medical therapy at 1 year (52% versus 25%) and 2 years (23% versus 8%). Additionally, the LVAD recipients' functional status was significantly better than that of the medical-therapy patients. Similarly, in a study comparing pneumatic HeartMate recipients with medical-therapy patients, the LVAD patients were more likely to survive to transplant (71% versus 36%, $P = .001$), and the LVAD recipients' functional capacity improved substantially after device implantation [5].

In addition to improving clinical outcomes, LVADs also seem to enhance QOL in patients who have HF. Patients interviewed before and 1 to 2 weeks after LVAD implantation report a substantial increase in their overall QOL and a decrease in overall symptom distress [6]. Additionally, in the REMATCH trial, scores on the physical-function and emotional-role subscales of the SF-36, Beck Depression Inventory scores, and NYHA class were all significantly better in the LVAD recipients than in the medical-therapy patients at 1 year. Minnesota Living with Heart Failure Questionnaire scores were also better in the LVAD group than in the medical-therapy group at 1 year, but the difference was not significant [3].

The new axial-flow LVADs have an even greater potential for improving QOL in patients

who have HF than conventional LVADs. Pumps such as the Jarvik 2000 (Jarvik Heart Inc., New York, New York) and the HeartMate II (Thoratec Corp.) are smaller and quieter than conventional LVADs because they use a simple continuous-flow technology rather than a pulsatile mechanism. The Jarvik is also virtually silent, and it does not produce the pulsing sensation that patients who have conventional LVADs sometimes find bothersome. Additionally, axial flow pumps have few moving parts, which should improve reliability and decrease mechanical failure rates.

Study findings indicate that QOL may improve dramatically in patients who have HF after implantation of the Jarvik 2000 [7,8]. The authors administered the Minnesota Living with Heart Failure Questionnaire immediately before implantation of the Jarvik 2000, 1 month after implantation, immediately before heart transplantation, and 1 month after transplantation [9]. One month after implantation of the device, the nine patients who completed the study showed significant improvements in physical ($P < .008$), emotional ($P < .02$), and overall QOL ($P < .008$). Although the implantation procedure is invasive and requires a substantial recovery period, patients reported better physical functioning 1 month after implantation than they did before the surgery. These findings suggest that the functional benefits conferred by the device outweigh the functional losses that patients experience in the postoperative period. Also, patients who had the device showed considerable functional gains and, in the first month after implantation, were able to walk further than before and perform more self-care activities without help [10]. These improvements were maintained until the device was explanted. Because there was no significant change in QOL between the end of LVAD support and 1 month after heart transplantation, it seems that LVAD support may be as good as heart transplantation in improving QOL.

However, LVADs may cause bleeding and thromboembolic complications, and infection is a particular concern during LVAD support. Patients who have conventional pulsatile LVADs are prone to infections [11,12]. In patients who had a mean duration of support of 106 ± 97 days (range 7–504 days), the incidence of infection was more than 40% [13]. Fortunately, during extended support, most infections occur at the driveline site and often can be easily resolved [14].

In the REMATCH trial, infection and mechanical failure of the device contributed importantly to the low 2-year survival rate of 23%. The device employed—the HeartMate XVE—requires a large percutaneous line, which can become a conduit for bacterial and fungal infection. Malnutrition was identified in these patients as a predisposing factor to infection and other complications. Factors contributing to postoperative malnutrition include early satiety, nausea, or both from the bulk of the implanted device; chronic inflammation associated with HF and the device; and severe and often-underdiagnosed preoperative debilitation [15].

Because these pumps are large, a substantial pump pocket must be formed around them, and the blood that collects in this pump pocket can be a culture medium for bacteria. The axial flow devices, on the other hand, are much smaller than conventional LVADs. Furthermore, the Jarvik 2000 is implanted within the left ventricle, eliminating the need for a pump pocket altogether. One study has shown that the Jarvik 2000 is associated with a lower infection rate than a conventional LVAD [7]. Additionally, the 26 patients in the authors' previously published clinical study experienced no significant device-related infections [10]. Because infections can reduce QOL by interfering with daily activities, requiring patients to take additional medications or necessitating a return to the hospital, the reduced infection rate associated with the Jarvik 2000 may enable the device to enhance QOL to a greater extent than conventional LVADs.

Mechanical failure of the LVAD was the second most frequent cause of death in the REMATCH trial's device group. The findings of inflow-valve failure and late erosions of the outflow graft resulting from kinking have already led to modifications in the device's design. Malfunction of the mechanical parts, such as rupture of the lining, motor failure, and wear on the bearings, also limits the durability of the device. Device failure limited use of the HeartMate XVE to 2 years or less. New devices have longer life spans, however; the Jarvik 2000 is expected to last 5 years.

One study suggests that patients survive longer after heart transplantation if they were supported by HeartMate XVE LVADs than if they did not have LVAD support during the waiting period [16]. However, patients supported by conventional LVADs also have greater cognitive impairment and are more likely to be unemployed 1 year after heart transplantation [17].

The authors recently evaluated the ease of use and reliability of the Jarvik device and the frequency of medical problems in outpatients with these pumps. There were no readmissions for technical reasons, and the pump never failed. QOL improved and was not adversely affected by the need to monitor or maintain the LVAS [18].

Cardiac support with an LVAD can significantly improve symptoms of HF and, in some cases, lead to complete recovery [19–22]. Signs of improvement in LVAD-supported patients include decreased levels of epinephrine, norepinephrine, angiotensin II, and arginine vasopressin, as well as interleukin-6, interleukin-8, and tissue necrosis factor-alpha [23–25]. Additionally, long-term LVAD support reduces collagen content and myocyte size in the myocardium and improves contractility and response to β-adrenergic stimulation, suggesting that prolonged cardiac unloading with the LVAD promotes reverse remodeling [26,27].

However, patient selection is important because LVAD support does not produce complete recovery in all patients who have HF [28]. The degree of irreversible myocardial damage at the time of LVAD implantation as well as the quality of medical management after implantation are important determinants of outcome after LVAD implantation [29].

Symptomatic relief with cardiac resynchronization therapy placement

In patients who have advanced HF and a prolonged QRS interval, CRT has been shown to improve symptoms and hemodynamics, increase exercise tolerance, and decrease the risk of death from any cause [30–33]. In the Multicenter InSync Randomized Clinical Evaluation (MIRACLE) study, CRT resulted in clinical improvement in patients who had moderate-to-severe HF (LVEF <35%) and an intraventricular conduction delay (QRS interval >130 msec) [33]. After 6 months, the 228 CRT patients could walk farther in 6 minutes and had greater endurance on the treadmill during exercise testing than the 225 patients in the control group. The CRT patients also had a greater decrease in LVEF, less need for hospitalization and intravenous medications, and greater improvement in NYHA class and QOL. However, 4 of the CRT patients had refractory hypotension, bradycardia, or asystole, and 2 of them died during implantation. Two other patients had perforation of the coronary sinus requiring peri-cardiocentesis. Also, implantation of the CRT device was unsuccessful in 8% of patients. These findings are similar to those of the Cardiac Resynchronization in Heart Failure study—the largest (813 patients) and longest-lasting (30 months) CRT study yet performed—in which echocardiography was used to confirm ventricular dyssynchrony, and which showed CRT-related reductions in morbidity and mortality in addition to aforementioned findings [32]. However, the rate of nonresponse to CRT was 40%.

The ability of CRT to relieve symptoms and improve exercise capacity and QOL in patients who have chronic HF is probably related to reverse remodeling of the left ventricle [33–35]. Significant reduction in mitral regurgitation and left ventricular mass, signs of reverse remodeling, was noted in the MIRACLE trial [33]. In the Pacing Therapies for Congestive Heart Failure (PATH-CHF) trial, left ventricular end-diastolic volumes were significantly smaller in patients who exhibited reverse remodeling when treated with biventricular pacing [35].

Approximately 18% to 52% of patients do not respond to CRT [30–32,36]. Also, the incidence of sudden cardiac death in patients who have CRT remains high [31]. The wide variation in clinical response rates among studies reflects a lack of consensus on the clinical criteria for sudden cardiac death. Identifying more and better predictors of sudden cardiac death and other outcomes after CRT could lead to better patient selection and could lower the nonresponse rate. To this end, there has been growing interest in identifying new markers for dyssynchrony and developing techniques to optimize device settings, as well as improving medical management [37–40].

Studies have used entry thresholds for QRS duration ranging from more than 120 ms in the MUltisite STimulation in cardiomyopathy trial to more than 150 ms in the COMPANION trial [31,41]. However, evidence that CRT may benefit patients who have HF with a "narrow" QRS calls into question the use of a specific QRS threshold to reveal ventricular dyssynchrony when selecting patients for CRT [42,43]. In 15% to 30% of patients who have HF, the regional delays in the electrical activation of myocardial masses cause dyssynchronous contraction of the left ventricle [44]. Standard ECG may not show the local changes in electrical activation, which may produce a vector that is too small to be detected. Therefore, in these patients, dyssynchronous ventricular contraction of the left ventricle can be present without changing the QRS interval on a standard surface ECG. Other, more sensitive diagnostic methods have been suggested that may better define the electrical dyssynchrony in HF; these include magnetic resonance imaging (although this alternative is relatively expensive) and echocardiography [38,42,45,46].

Mechanical dyssynchrony, defined as an electromechanical delay on tissue Doppler echocardiography imaging, has been found in up to 50% of patients who have HF with normal surface QRS [47,48]. However, this technology is still relatively expensive, operator-dependent, and not available in all diagnostic laboratories.

Recently, scientists at the National Aeronautics and Space Administration (NASA) developed a high-frequency QRS electrocardiograph that allows the analysis of the otherwise invisible high frequencies (150–250 Hz) present within the QRS complex [49]. High-frequency QRS analysis is a fully automated, simple noninvasive technique that can be easily implemented with conventional ECG equipment [50]. The authors are using this method to better define electrical dyssynchrony in patients who have HF (NYHA class III, ejection fraction <40%) and a QRS interval 130 msec or less on a standard surface ECG. If further studies confirm its ability to detect mechanical dyssynchrony, high-frequency QRS analysis will help clinicians identify patients who have HF who would benefit from CRT.

The reverse remodeling induced by CRT could reduce neurohormonal activity, in addition to improving anatomic and functional parameters. Indeed, studies have shown significant reductions in brain natriuretic peptide (BNP) levels after 4 to 6 days of continuous biventricular pacing, as well as after long-term CRT [32,51–53]. These studies also have found a positive correlation between clinical improvement and BNP levels after biventricular pacing, and BNP measurement seems to be useful for monitoring the efficacy of CRT. In one study, withdrawing CRT raised BNP levels, which decreased again when CRT was restarted in patients who had undergone it for longer than 6 months [54]. Levels of BNP correlated with the degree of left ventricular reverse remodeling and improvement in exercise capacity.

When the authors analyzed clinical, ECG, echocardiographic, and laboratory data recorded at baseline and after 3 months of CRT treatment, they, too, found that BNP might be a useful prognostic indicator in patients treated with CRT

[55]. It seems that increases in BNP levels may be early markers of CRT nonresponse even before major clinical decompensation occurs. Patients who do not show any significant response to CRT should be considered for earlier treatment with LVAD or transplant.

Previously, the authors have found that prolonged QTc interval predicts mortality—particularly sudden cardiac death—in patients who have advanced HF and high BNP levels [56]. The results of recent preclinical and clinical studies suggest that CRT is associated with QTc interval prolongation and that polymorphic ventricular tachycardia may represent a potential complication of CRT [57,58]. Patients who have CRT-induced QTc interval prolongation are probably not good candidates for this therapy. Again, LVAD implantation, which leads to QTc interval shortening, may be a viable treatment alternative in these patients [59,60].

Further efforts to improve CRT may result in better, more individualized treatment options. One promising method is sequential ventricular pacing, a newer therapeutic method of adjusting the difference in pace between the ventricles to produce a nearly equal delay.

Summary

Evidence suggests that the circulatory support provided by LVADs substantially improves QOL for patients who have HF. Implantation of LVADs has become an established treatment, both as a bridge to heart transplantation and as destination therapy in patients who are not candidates for heart transplantation and are refractory to all medical treatment. In both types of patients, LVAD implantation is considered a better option for definitive treatment than is pharmacologic therapy. Data suggest that early LVAD implantation, before end-stage HF develops, is critical to slowing or reversing disease progression. Similarly, in indicated patients who have less advanced disease, CRT may be particularly beneficial.

Future studies should compare the relative impact of pulsatile and axial flow LVADs on QOL. It would also be valuable to examine the long-term effects of the LVAD on QOL in patients who receive the device as destination therapy rather than as a bridge to transplant.

In conclusion, despite the ease of placement and the low risks associated with CRT devices, there is a need to clearly identify the subset of patients who have advanced HF who will benefit most from this therapy. This would prevent giving false hope to this subset of patients and would allow for the timely implementation of more definitive therapies (ie, LVAD implantation or heart transplantation). The future will see LVADs that can be implanted in a catheterization lab, with much lower procedural morbidity and mortality, and it is likely these pumps will be used synergistically with CRT devices.

Acknowledgment

Stephen N. Palmer, PhD, ELS, provided editorial support.

References

[1] McMurray JJ, Stewart S. Epidemiology, aetiology, and prognosis of heart failure. Heart 2000;83(5): 596–602.

[2] O'Connell JB, Bristow MR. Economic impact of heart failure in the United States: time for a different approach. J Heart Lung Transplant 1994;13(4): S107–12.

[3] Rose EA, Gelijns AC, Moskowitz AJ, et al. Long-term use of a left ventricular assist device for end-stage heart failure. N Engl J Med 2001;345(20): 1435–43.

[4] Hobbs FD, Kenkre JE, Roalfe AK, et al. Impact of heart failure and left ventricular systolic dysfunction on quality of life: a cross-sectional study comparing common chronic cardiac and medical disorders and a representative adult population. Eur Heart J 2002; 23(23):1867–76.

[5] Frazier OH, Rose EA, McCarthy P, et al. Improved mortality and rehabilitation of transplant candidates treated with a long-term implantable left ventricular assist system. Ann Surg 1995;222(3):327–36.

[6] Grady KL, Meyer P, Mattea A, et al. Improvement in quality of life outcomes 2 weeks after left ventricular assist device implantation. J Heart Lung Transplant 2001;20(6):657–69.

[7] Siegenthaler MP, Martin J, Pernice K, et al. The Jarvik 2000 is associated with less infections than the HeartMate left ventricular assist device. Eur J Cardiothorac Surg 2003;23(5):748–54.

[8] Westaby S, Banning AP, Saito S, et al. Circulatory support for long-term treatment of heart failure: experience with an intraventricular continuous flow pump. Circulation 2002;105(22):2588–91.

[9] Miller K, Myers TJ, Robertson K, et al. Quality of life in bridge-to-transplant patients with chronic heart failure after implantation of an axial flow ventricular assist device. Congest Heart Fail 2004; 10(5):226–9.

[10] Frazier OH, Myers TJ, Westaby S, et al. Use of the Jarvik 2000 left ventricular assist system as a bridge to heart transplantation or as destination therapy for patients with chronic heart failure. Ann Surg 2003; 237(5):631–6.

[11] Frazier OH, Rose EA, Oz MC, et al. Multicenter clinical evaluation of the HeartMate vented electric left ventricular assist system in patients awaiting heart transplantation. J Thorac Cardiovasc Surg 2001;122(6):1186–95.

[12] Argenziano M, Catanese KA, Moazami N, et al. The influence of infection on survival and successful transplantation in patients with left ventricular assist devices. J Heart Lung Transplant 1997;16(8):822–31.

[13] Wasler A, Springer E, Radovancevic B, et al. A comparison between intraperitoneal and extraperitoneal left ventricular assist system placement. ASAIO J 1996;42(5):M573–6.

[14] Pennington DG, McBride LR, Peigh PS, et al. Eight years' experience with bridging to cardiac transplantation. J Thorac Cardiovasc Surg 1994;107 (2):472–80.

[15] el-Amir NG, Gardocki M, Levin HR, et al. Gastrointestinal consequences of left ventricular assist device placement. ASAIO J 1996;42(3):150–3.

[16] Aaronson KD, Eppinger MJ, Dyke DB, et al. Left ventricular assist device therapy improves utilization of donor hearts. J Am Coll Cardiol 2002;39(8): 1247–54.

[17] Dew MA, Kormos RL, Winowich S, et al. Quality of life outcomes after heart transplantation in individuals bridged to transplant with ventricular assist devices. J Heart Lung Transplant 2001;20(11): 1199–212.

[18] Mesina HS, Myers TJ, Radovancevic B, et al. Patient management of a ventricular assist system after hospital discharge [abstract]. ASAIO J 2006; 52(2):59.

[19] Frazier OH. First use of an untethered, vented electric left ventricular assist device for long-term support. Circulation 1994;89(6):2908–14.

[20] Frazier OH, Myers TJ. Left ventricular assist system as a bridge to myocardial recovery. Ann Thorac Surg 1999;68(2):734–41.

[21] Hetzer R, Muller JH, Weng Y, et al. Bridging-to-recovery. Ann Thorac Surg 2001;71(Suppl 3): S109–13.

[22] Westaby S, Coats AJ. Mechanical bridge to myocardial recovery. Eur Heart J 1998;19(4):541–7.

[23] Goldstein DJ, Moazami N, Seldomridge JA, et al. Circulatory resuscitation with left ventricular assist device support reduces interleukins 6 and 8 levels. Ann Thorac Surg 1997;63(4):971–4.

[24] James KB, McCarthy PM, Thomas JD, et al. Effect of the implantable left ventricular assist device on neuroendocrine activation in heart failure. Circulation 1995;92(Suppl 9):II191–5.

[25] Torre-Amione G, Stetson SJ, Youker KA, et al. Decreased expression of tumor necrosis factor-alpha in failing human myocardium after mechanical circulatory support: a potential mechanism for cardiac recovery. Circulation 1999;100(11):1189–93.

[26] Bruckner BA, Stetson SJ, Perez-Verdia A, et al. Regression of fibrosis and hypertrophy in failing myocardium following mechanical circulatory support. J Heart Lung Transplant 2001;20(4): 457–64.

[27] Dipla K, Mattiello JA, Jeevanandam V, et al. Myocyte recovery after mechanical circulatory support in humans with end-stage heart failure. Circulation 1998;97(23):2316–22.

[28] Mancini DM, Beniaminovitz A, Levin H, et al. Low incidence of myocardial recovery after left ventricular assist device implantation in patients with chronic heart failure. Circulation 1998;98(22): 2383–9.

[29] Williams MR, Oz MC. Indications and patient selection for mechanical ventricular assistance. Ann Thorac Surg 2001;71(Suppl 3):S86–91.

[30] Abraham WT, Fisher WG, Smith AL, et al. Cardiac resynchronization in chronic heart failure. N Engl J Med 2002;346(24):1845–53.

[31] Bristow MR, Saxon LA, Boehmer J, et al. Cardiac-resynchronization therapy with or without an implantable defibrillator in advanced chronic heart failure. N Engl J Med 2004;350(21):2140–50.

[32] Cleland JG, Daubert JC, Erdmann E, et al. The effect of cardiac resynchronization on morbidity and mortality in heart failure. N Engl J Med 2005; 352(15):1539–49.

[33] Young JB, Abraham WT, Smith AL, et al. Combined cardiac resynchronization and implantable cardioversion defibrillation in advanced chronic heart failure: the MIRACLE ICD Trial. JAMA 2003;289(20):2685–94.

[34] Saxon LA, De Marco T, Schafer J, et al. Effects of long-term biventricular stimulation for resynchronization on echocardiographic measures of remodeling. Circulation 2002;105(11):1304–10.

[35] Stellbrink C, Breithardt OA, Franke A, et al. Impact of cardiac resynchronization therapy using hemodynamically optimized pacing on left ventricular remodeling in patients with congestive heart failure and ventricular conduction disturbances. J Am Coll Cardiol 2001;38(7):1957–65.

[36] Reuter S, Garrigue S, Barold SS, et al. Comparison of characteristics in responders versus nonresponders with biventricular pacing for drug-resistant congestive heart failure. Am J Cardiol 2002;89(3):346–50.

[37] Bax JJ, Ansalone G, Breithardt OA, et al. Echocardiographic evaluation of cardiac resynchronization therapy: ready for routine clinical use? A critical appraisal. J Am Coll Cardiol 2004;44(1): 1–9.

[38] Bax JJ, Marwick TH, Molhoek SG, et al. Left ventricular dyssynchrony predicts benefit of cardiac resynchronization therapy in patients with end-stage

heart failure before pacemaker implantation. Am J Cardiol 2003;92(10):1238–40.

[39] Doshi RN. Optimizing resynchronization therapy: can we increase the number of true responders? J Cardiovasc Electrophysiol 2005;16(Suppl 1):S48–51.

[40] Yu CM, Fung WH, Lin H, et al. Predictors of left ventricular reverse remodeling after cardiac resynchronization therapy for heart failure secondary to idiopathic dilated or ischemic cardiomyopathy. Am J Cardiol 2003;91(6):684–8.

[41] Linde C, Leclercq C, Rex S, et al. Long-term benefits of biventricular pacing in congestive heart failure: results from the MUltisite STimulation in cardiomyopathy (MUSTIC) study. J Am Coll Cardiol 2002;40(1):111–8.

[42] Achilli A, Sassara M, Ficili S, et al. Long-term effectiveness of cardiac resynchronization therapy in patients with refractory heart failure and "narrow" QRS. J Am Coll Cardiol 2003;42(12):2117–24.

[43] Turner MS, Bleasdale RA, Mumford CE, et al. Left ventricular pacing improves haemodynamic variables in patients with heart failure with a normal QRS duration. Heart 2004;90(5):502–5.

[44] Abraham WT. Cardiac resynchronization therapy for heart failure: biventricular pacing and beyond. Curr Opin Cardiol 2002;17(4):346–52.

[45] Helm RH, Leclercq C, Faris OP, et al. Cardiac dyssynchrony analysis using circumferential versus longitudinal strain: implications for assessing cardiac resynchronization. Circulation 2005;111(21):2760–7.

[46] Pitzalis MV, Iacoviello M, Romito R, et al. Cardiac resynchronization therapy tailored by echocardiographic evaluation of ventricular asynchrony. J Am Coll Cardiol 2002;40(9):1615–22.

[47] Bleeker GB, Schalij MJ, Molhoek SG, et al. Relationship between QRS duration and left ventricular dyssynchrony in patients with end-stage heart failure. J Cardiovasc Electrophysiol 2004;15(5):544–9.

[48] Yu CM, Lin H, Zhang Q, et al. High prevalence of left ventricular systolic and diastolic asynchrony in patients with congestive heart failure and normal QRS duration. Heart 2003;89(1):54–60.

[49] Schlegel TT, Kulecz WB, DePalma JL, et al. Real-time 12-lead high-frequency QRS electrocardiography for enhanced detection of myocardial ischemia and coronary artery disease. Mayo Clin Proc 2004; 79(3):339–50.

[50] Delgado RM III, Poulin GV, Vrtovec B, et al. The utility of high frequency QRS electrocardiogram in the diagnosis of cardiomyopathy. J Am Coll Cardiol 2004;43(5 Suppl 1):208A–9A.

[51] Erol-Yilmaz A, Verberne HJ, Schrama TA, et al. Cardiac resynchronization induces favorable neurohumoral changes. Pacing Clin Electrophysiol 2005; 28(4):304–10.

[52] Filzmaier K, Sinha AM, Breithardt OA, et al. Short-term effects of cardiac resynchronization on brain natriuretic peptide release in patients with systolic heart failure and ventricular conduction disturbance. J Am Coll Cardiol 2006;39(Suppl 1):S111.

[53] Hernandez Madrid A, Miguelanez Diaz M, Escobar Cervantes C, et al. [Usefulness of brain natriuretic peptide to evaluate patients with heart failure treated with cardiac resynchronization]. Rev Esp Cardiol 2004;57(4):299–305.

[54] Sinha AM, Filzmaier K, Breithardt OA, et al. Usefulness of brain natriuretic peptide release as a surrogate marker of the efficacy of long-term cardiac resynchronization therapy in patients with heart failure. Am J Cardiol 2003;91(6):755–8.

[55] Delgado RM, Palanichamy N, Radovancevic R, et al. Brain natriuretic peptide levels and response to cardiac resynchronization therapy in heart failure patients. Congest Heart Fail 2006;12(5):250–3.

[56] Vrtovec B, Delgado R, Zewail A, et al. Prolonged QTc interval and high B-type natriuretic peptide levels together predict mortality in patients with advanced heart failure. Circulation 2003;107(13):1764–9.

[57] Medina-Ravell VA, Lankipalli RS, Yan GX, et al. Effect of epicardial or biventricular pacing to prolong QT interval and increase transmural dispersion of repolarization: does resynchronization therapy pose a risk for patients predisposed to long QT or torsade de pointes? Circulation 2003;107(5):740–6.

[58] Fish JM, Di Diego JM, Nesterenko V, et al. Epicardial activation of left ventricular wall prolongs QT interval and transmural dispersion of repolarization: implications for biventricular pacing. Circulation 2004;109(17):2136–42.

[59] Harding JD, Piacentino V III, Gaughan JP, et al. Electrophysiological alterations after mechanical circulatory support in patients with advanced cardiac failure. Circulation 2001;104(11):1241–7.

[60] Xydas S, Rosen RS, Ng C, et al. Mechanical unloading leads to echocardiographic, electrocardiographic, neurohormonal, and histologic recovery. J Heart Lung Transplant 2006;25(1):7–15.

ELSEVIER
SAUNDERS

Heart Failure Clin 3 (2007) 267–273

HEART
FAILURE
CLINICS

Should Patients who have Persistent Severe Symptoms Receive a Left Ventricular Assist Device or Cardiac Resynchronization Therapy as the Next Step?

John Cleland, MD, FESC, FACC*, Ahmed Tageldien, MSc, MD, Olga Khaleva, MD, Neil Hobson, MBBS, Andrew L. Clark, MD

University of Hull, Castle Hill Hospital, Kingston-upon-Hull, UK

Many patients who have heart failure experience severe recurrent or persistent symptoms despite standard pharmacologic treatment with diuretics, ACE inhibitors or angiotensin receptor blockers, aldosterone antagonists, and beta-blockers [1–3]. Careful review of standard medication may identify that the dose of one or more components is not optimal and can be adjusted for greater effect. Finding the optimal dose and combination of diuretics may be particularly difficult. Excessive doses will cause hypotension, renal dysfunction, and worsening symptoms. Insufficient doses will also lead to worsening symptoms. Digoxin probably still has a role for the management of advanced symptoms, especially when the patient has atrial fibrillation, because beta-blockers often do not adequately control ventricular rate [4]. Correction of anemia with iron supplements when it is due to iron deficiency or erythropoietin-stimulating peptides when not due to specific haematinic deficiency may also improve symptoms, although the data are not robust [5]. Withdrawal of nonsteroidal anti-inflammatory drugs, including aspirin, also seems to reduce the need for hospitalization for worsening heart failure [6,7]. However, when standard pharmacologic therapy has failed, surgical and device options should be considered.

Two substantial studies are underway to assess the benefits of revascularization with or without the benefits of surgical left ventricular remodeling [8–10]. Currently there is no evidence that revascularization of patients who have heart failure and LVSD is safe or effective, even when a large amount of viable but hibernating myocardium is present. We should obtain the first results of trials in 2007. Revascularization is not discussed further in this manuscript.

The initial enthusiasm for skeletal myoblast and stem cell transplantation into the failing myocardium has been tempered by experience. There is now considerable uncertainty whether this approach provides worthwhile benefits [11,12]. Hopefully, refinements in the technologic approach might improve results.

The two surgical technologies that have shown benefit on symptoms and survival are left ventricular assist devices (LVADs) and cardiac resynchronization therapy (CRT), with or without a defibrillator function [3,13–15]. The purpose of this manuscript is to describe the benefits of CRT and the gaps in our knowledge that are an impediment to clinical practice and may be exploited by further research and then to compare that to what we know about LVADs. However, it should be clear from the outset that there is a role for both in the management of advanced heart failure.

Cardiac dyssynchrony

Cardiac dyssynchrony is conceptually simple but rather difficult to define and measure on an individual patient basis [13]. Indeed, it may not be

* Corresponding author. University of Hull, Castle Hill Hospital, Kingston-upon-Hull, HU 16 5JQ, UK.
E-mail address: j.g.cleland@hull.ac.uk (J. Cleland).

1551-7136/07/$ - see front matter © 2007 Elsevier Inc. All rights reserved.
doi:10.1016/j.hfc.2007.05.005

heartfailure.theclinics.com

worth measuring in clinical practice because it may be a near universal accompaniment of LVSD. The issue may not be whether dyssynchrony is present or absent, but rather how much of each of the six or seven different types of dyssynchrony is present.

Cardiac dyssynchrony means that one or more parts of the heart do not contract in an optimal sequence. This can mean that atrioventricular conduction is prolonged, leading to diastolic mitral regurgitation. Alternatively, it can mean that some parts of the left ventricular wall contract late. This leads to myocardial contraction expending much of its energy to move the opposing myocardium that has either not started to contract or already begun to relax resulting in a change in shape of the ventricle but little effective ejection of blood. This can be circumferential or longitudinal. Importantly, contraction that is present but delayed needs to be distinguished from akinetic or passively moving areas of myocardial scar. If the left ventricle is affected by dyssynchrony, then usually there will also be interventricular dyssynchrony. If the papillary muscle is affected by dyssynchrony, then there will be mitral regurgitation. Each type of dyssynchrony is probably deleterious and will vary heterogeneously amongst patients. Various physiologic stresses can cause or exacerbate dyssynchrony in hearts that show little dyssynchrony at rest. Because important dyssynchrony may reflect differences of a few tens of milliseconds in the timing of heart contraction, it can be difficult to measure.

Confused? You should be and so are many of the investigators in this area. Indeed, those who organized the large outcome trials had so little confidence in cardiac imaging that they used the QRS duration greater than 120 msec on the surface ECG rather than the echocardiogram as a marker of dyssynchrony. Only the Cardiac Resynchronization–Heart Failure (CARE-HF) trial used echo markers of dyssynchrony as part of the inclusion criteria for the small group of patients who had QRS 120 to 149 msec [16]. People have assumed that because prolonged QRS duration is a marker of a worse prognosis and a higher prevalence of dyssynchrony on echocardiography, that dyssynchrony itself confers an adverse prognosis. However, QRS duration is also a rough guide to left ventricular ejection fraction, and this could be the link between QRS duration and prognosis [17]. Finally, the few data that exist suggest that echocardiographically measured dyssynchrony is an independent predictor *of a better prognosis* once corrected for ejection fraction, possibly because it is a sign of a greater extent of viable myocardium [13].

The effects of cardiac resynchronization therapy

More than 3000 patients have participated in at least eight randomized controlled trials published so far (Table 1) [18]. Three of these were conducted double blind and are therefore a robust test of symptoms. Each trial showed that approximately one third of the control group improved substantially, presumably in response to intensification of medical care or a placebo response. Another third improved with CRT but not in the control group, and the remainder had little response in either group. Presumably a few patients might have been made worse by CRT, but few reports of the effects of switching off CRT in deteriorating patients exist. Worsening in such patients may reflect changes in the underlying disease rather than the effects of intervention. In the clinic, this means that approximately two thirds of patients may be expected to get symptomatic improvement with CRT. This is accompanied by improvements in ventricular function; a reduction in mitral regurgitation; an increase in systolic blood pressure, which is usually low in this population; and an increase in exercise capacity [3,13].

In the CARE-HF study, CRT reduced the rate of hospitalization for worsening heart failure by approximately half, a large effect compared with pharmacologic therapy [3]. CRT reduced all-cause mortality by 40% over 3 years; thus, more patients were kept alive and were therefore at risk of hospitalization [14]. The reduction in mortality was due to a reduction in sudden death and worsening heart failure by roughly similar amounts. There did not seem to be a strong relationship between the effects of CRT on symptoms and its effects on morbidity and mortality. In other words, the "mantra" that one third of patients do not respond to CRT may be misleading and will only apply if the criteria for response is restricted to an improvement in symptoms. However, CRT is probably at least as effective in preventing deterioration as it is at making people feel better, and this cannot be assessed accurately in observational trials but requires randomized trials that describe outcome in a control group.

There are many reasons why patients might not appear to respond well to CRT, including inadequate deployment or programming of the device, the amount and site of myocardial scar, noncardiovascular comorbidity, intervening events, rehabilitation and psychologic factors. In summary, the statement that 30% of patients do not respond to CRT is naïve and misleading.

Who should get cardiac resynchronization therapy?

Despite the complexity of the substrate, atrio-biventricular pacing, a crude intervention has been shown to have large benefits in patients that have been selected using only ECG criteria.

Observational studies suggest a link between dyssynchrony measured by echocardiography and the benefits of CRT but cannot distinguish between the natural history of the disease and the effect of intervention. In other words, patients who are destined to do well will do well whether or not they get CRT. Only randomized trials can show who benefits from intervention because they have a control group that informs the observer of how well or badly the patient would have done without CRT. Randomized controlled trials suggest a weak association between the effects of CRT on mortality and dyssynchrony that probably explains no more than 25% of the benefit of CRT. It is less clear whether dyssynchrony predicts the short-term effect of CRT on symptoms.

There are few data on the effects of CRT in patients who have less severe symptoms. The analyses conducted so far suggest that there may be mortality and morbidity benefits even in patients who do not have severe symptoms [13].

Patients who have more severe mitral regurgitation have a generally worse prognosis and perhaps a more striking response to CRT, although this effect disappears on multivariate analysis. This might reflect a selective additional benefit of CRT amongst patients who have moderate to severe mitral regurgitation. In contrast, patients who have below median plasma concentrations of NT-proBNP tend to have a greater benefit from CRT, suggesting that there may be a point at which cardiac dysfunction is so severe that the effects of CRT diminish [14].

Accordingly, if little of the benefit of CRT can be explained by the severity of symptoms or the amount of dyssynchrony measured at rest, then why should CRT be restricted to patients who have dyssynchrony and advanced symptoms? There are also strong arguments for implanting

CRT- defibrillator rather than an implantable cardiac defibrillator (ICD) in all patients who have LVSD, because many of these patients will develop a broad QRS and/or dyssynchrony during follow-up [13], and all patients who have LVSD should receive biventricular pacing if they require ventricular pacing for an atrioventricular conduction disorder. These arguments will be better informed by the results of ongoing clinical trials [19]. ICDs are not cost-effective when used for primary prevention in patients who have heart failure and a poor prognosis. Only patients who are expected to survive 5 to 10 years, assuming that sudden death is prevented, should be chosen for such an intervention [20]. The problem with choosing patients who need an ICD is finding patients who neither have too good nor too bad a prognosis to warrant intervention.

Left ventricular assist devices

Conceptually, LVADs should improve cardiac function regardless of the cause of dysfunction. Small devices that provide only partial support appear able to offer substantial benefit in experimental models.

In contrast to CRT, there is a paucity of evidence from adequately controlled trials showing benefit. One substantial trial exists that showed that LVADs could improve survival, although outcome in control and intervention groups was exceedingly poor [15]. It is likely that the population was so sick that the result was inevitable. LVADs seemed to reduce the risk of dying of heart failure dramatically, but this was replaced by an increased risk of dying from infection or thromboembolic complications. The procedural mortality for LVADs is much higher than for CRT. The cost is also higher. For all these reasons, at this moment, CRT is the preferred option whenever feasible. Further randomized trials are required to determine whether there is any substantial population where CRT is ineffective and in which patient LVADs might be the better option. The development of safe, low-cost, low-maintenance, easily implanted LVADs seems likely and could well change this balance. There may come a time when patients are selected for an LVAD or CRT depending on their clinical features, and it is not impossible that LVADs could become the dominant therapy in due course. However, this seems unlikely in the near term. For the moment, the lucky and

Table 1
Published randomized controlled trials of cardiac resynchronization therapy

Study	n	Type	Pacing mode	Inclusion criteria				Main results
				NYHA Class	EF (%)	LVEDD (mm)	QRS duration (msec)	
MUSTIC	67	Crossover	BiV-CRT	III	<35	>60	>150	Improvement in 6MWT NYHA functional class QOL, peak VO2, LV volumes, MR, less hospitalizations
MUSTIC-AF	41	Single blind	CRT on versus off with VVI back-up 70bpm	III	<35	>60	>200 (RV paced)	Improvement in 6MWT NYHA functional class QOL, peak VO2, LV volumes, MR, less hospitalizations
MIRACLE	453	Parallel-arm	BiV-CRT	III–IV	35	≥55	≥130	Improvement in 6MWT NYHA functional class QOL, LVEF LVEDD, MR
MIRACLE ICD	369	Parallel arm	CRT-D versus ICD	III–IV	35	≥55	≥130	Improvement in NYHA functional class, QOL

Study	N	Design	Comparison	NYHA	EF		QRS	Outcomes/measures
MIRACLE-ICD-II	186	Double-Blind parallel arm	CRT on v off	II	<35	≥55	≥130	Peak VO2, VE/CO2, NYHA class, QOL, 6-min walk distance, LV volumes and ejection fraction, and composite clinical response
CONTAK CD/VENTAK CHF	490	Crossover	CRT-D versus ICD	II–IV	35	Median 71	120	Improvement in 6MWT NYHA functional class QOL LVEF, LV volumes
COMPANION	1520	Parallel arm	CRT-D versus CRT versus control	III–IV	35	Median 67	120	Reduced all-cause mortality/ hospitalization
CARE-HF	813	Parallel-arm	BiV-CRT	III–IV	35	>30 mm/m (height)	120–149 + interventricular dyssynchrony or 150+	Reduced mortality/ morbidity; improvement in NYHA functional class QOL, LVEF, LVESV

Abbreviations: 6MWT, 6-minute walk test; BiV, biventricular; CHF, chronic heart failure; COMPANION, The Comparison of Medical, Pacing, and Defibrillator Therapies in Heart Failure trial; CRT, cardiac resynchronisation; CRT-D, CRT with a defibrillator function; MUSTIC, Multisite Stimulation in Cardiomyopathies trial in patients in sinus rhythm; MUSTIC-AF, Multisite Stimulation in Cardiomyopathies trial in patients with atrial firbrillation.

determined few might consider migrating from CRT or CRT-defibrillator therapy to an LVAD if they get an insufficient response to the former. Finding out which patients truly do not respond to CRT and why are matters of some urgency [13].

Meanwhile, there will be further pharmacologic advances in the management of heart failure. Some of these will threaten to replace device therapy, but many will be used either in synergy with devices or when devices have failed to give an adequate or sustained response. The development of intelligent, diagnostic implantable devices is an exciting development that will open up many new therapeutic opportunities [21].

References

[1] Cleland JGF, Swedberg K, Follath F, et al. For the study group on diagnosis of the working group on heart failure of the European society of cardiology. The EuroHeart failure survey programme: survey on the quality of care among patients with heart failure in Europe. Part 1: patient characteristics and diagnosis. Eur Heart J 2003;24:422–63.

[2] Cleland JGF, Cohen-Solal A, Cosin-Aguilar J, et al. For the IMPROVEMENT of Heart Failure Programme Committees and Investigators and the Study Group on Diagnosis of the Working Group on Heart Failure of the European Society of Cardiology. An International Survey of the Management of Heart Failure in Primary Care. The IMPROVEMENT of Heart Failure Programme. Lancet 2002; 360:1631–9.

[3] Cleland JGF, Daubert J-C, Erdmann E, et al. For the Cardiac Resynchronisation - Heart Failure (CARE-HF) Study Investigators. The effect of cardiac resynchronization on morbidity and mortality in heart failure. N Engl J Med 2005;352:1539–49.

[4] Khand AU, Rankin AC, Martin W, et al. Carvedilol alone or in combination with digoxin for the management of atrial fibrillation in patients with heart failure. J Am Coll Cardiol 2003;42:1944–51.

[5] Ponikowski P, Anker S, Szachniewicz J, et al. Effect of darbepoetin alfa on exercise tolerance in anemic patients with symptomatic chronic heart failure: a randomized, double-blind, placebo-controlled trial. J Am Coll Cardiol 2007;49:753–62.

[6] Cleland JGF, Ghosh J, Freemantle N, et al. Clinical trials update and cumulative meta-analyses from the American College of Cardiology: WATCH, SCD-HeFT, DINAMIT, CASINO, INSPIRE, STRATUS-US, RIO-LIPIDS and cardiac resynchronisation therapy in heart failure. Eur J Heart Fail 2004;6:501–8.

[7] Cleland JGF, Findlay I, Jafri S, et al. The Warfarin/ Aspirin Study in Heart Failure (WASH): a randomized trial comparing antithrombotic strategies for patients with heart failure. Am Heart J 2004;148: 157–64.

[8] Cleland JGF, Freemantle N, Ball SG, et al. The heart failure revascularization trial (HEART): rationale design and methodology. Eur J Heart Fail 2003; 5(3):295–303.

[9] Buckberg GD. Questions and answers about the STICH trial: a different perspective. J Thorac Cardiovasc Surg 2005;130:245–9.

[10] Cleland JGF, Alamgir F, Nikitin N, et al. What is the optimal medical management of ischaemic heart failure? Prog Cardiovasc Dis 2001;43(5):433–55.

[11] Schachinger V, Erbs S, Elsasser A, et al. Improved clinical outcome after intracoronary administration of bone-marrow-derived progenitor cells in acute myocardial infarction: final 1-year results of the REPAIR-AMI trial. Eur Heart J 2006;27: 2775–83.

[12] Bartunek J, Dimmeler S, Drexler H, et al. The consensus of the task force of the European society of cardiology concerning the clinical investigation of the use of autologous adult stem cells for repair of the heart. Eur Heart J 2006;27:1338–40.

[13] Cleland JGF, Nasir M, Tageldien A. Cardiac resynchronization therapy or atriobiventricular pacing—what should it be called? Nat Clin Pract Cardiovasc Med 2007;4(2):90–101.

[14] Cleland JGF, Daubert J-C, Erdmann E, et al. On behalf of the CARE-HF study investigators. Longer-term effects of cardiac resynchronization therapy on mortality in heart failure [the Cardiac Resynchronization - Heart Failure (CARE-HF) trial extension phase]. Eur Heart J 2006;27(16): 1928–32.

[15] Rose EA, Gelijns AC, Moskowitz AJ, et al. Long-term mechanical left ventricular assistance for end-stage heart failure. N Engl J Med 2001;345: 1435–43.

[16] Cleland JGF, Daubert JC, Erdmann E, et al. Design and methodology of the CARE-HF trial. A randomised trial of cardiac resynchronisation in patients with heart failure and ventricular dyssynchrony. Eur J Heart Fail 2001;3:481–9.

[17] Khan NK, Goode KM, Cleland JGF, et al. For the EuroHeart failure survey investigators. Prevalence of ECG abnormalities in an international survey of patients with suspected or confirmed heart failure at death or discharge. Eur J Heart Fail 2007;9: 491–501.

[18] Freemantle N, Tharmanathan P, Calvert MJ, et al. Cardiac resynchronization for patients with heart failure due to left ventricular systolic dysfunction a systematic review and meta-analysis. Eur J Heart Fail 2006;8:433–40.

[19] Moss AJ, Brown MW, Cannom DS, et al. Multicenter automatic defibrillator implantation trial-cardiac resynchronization therapy (MADIT-CRT): design and clinical protocol. Ann Noninvasive Electrocardiol 2005;10:34–43.

[20] Yao G, Freemantle N, Calvert M, et al. The long-term cost-effectiveness of cardiac resynchronization therapy with or without an implantable cardioverter-defibrillator. Eur Heart J 2007;28(1): 42–51.

[21] Cleland JGF. The Trans-European Network - Home-Care Management System (TEN-HMS) Study: an investigation of the effect of telemedicine on outcomes in Europe. Dis Manag Health Out 2006;14(Suppl 1):23–8.

ELSEVIER
SAUNDERS

Heart Failure Clin 3 (2007) 275–288

Does Myectomy Convey Survival Benefit in Hypertrophic Cardiomyopathy?

Anna Woo, MD, SM, FRCPC, FACC*,
Harry Rakowski, MD, FRCPC, FACC

University of Toronto, Toronto, ON, Canada

Hypertrophic cardiomyopathy (HCM) is a complex disorder and concepts regarding this condition have evolved considerably since its modern description in the 1950s [1,2]. Although once perceived as a rare disease causing sudden cardiac death (SCD) in young adults [2], HCM is now recognized as a relatively common genetic disorder affecting 1 in 500 individuals and characterized by a wide spectrum of clinical manifestations [3,4]. Dynamic left ventricular outflow tract (LVOT) obstruction has been a prominent aspect of HCM and, in the early years of the disease's recognition, its presence was inextricably linked to the diagnosis of this condition [5,6]. Patients who have the obstructive form of HCM have unique and distinguishing clinical and hemodynamic features [4–6].

The dynamic LVOT obstruction of HCM has generated much interest and controversy; its existence, cause, diagnosis, treatment, and prognosis have all provoked debate [3,4]. Aside from its hemodynamic effects, some investigators had questioned the importance of obstruction and regarded it as a secondary finding in this disease [7,8]. Multiple echocardiographic and hemodynamic studies support the view that LVOT obstruction is caused by systolic anterior motion (SAM) of the anterior mitral leaflet, contact of the mitral leaflet with the hypertrophied interventricular septum, and consequent obstruction to

blood flow in the outflow tract during systole [3,4,9]. LVOT obstruction is accompanied by mitral regurgitation [10,11], and these lesions are largely responsible for the disabling symptoms (eg, dyspnea, angina, presyncope, syncope) and hemodynamic abnormalities associated with obstructive HCM [3,4,6]. The presence of an LVOT gradient measuring at least 30 mm Hg is generally accepted as the definition for obstructive HCM [3].

At the present time there is a general consensus that patients who have symptoms attributable to LVOT obstruction should receive treatment to diminish or abolish the LVOT gradient [3]. Treatment options include medications (negative inotropic agents), dual chamber (DDD) permanent pacing, septal ethanol ablation (SEA), or surgical myectomy. All of these therapies have variable effects on reducing symptoms and on controlling the LVOT gradient [3,4]. The longest experience has been with surgery, which was first performed in this condition in the late 1950s [5]. Because myectomy has consistently improved symptoms and LVOT obstruction, many investigators regard this procedure as the optimum treatment of obstructive HCM [3,12]. Myectomy remains controversial, however, because it is unclear if there is a survival advantage with myectomy compared with conservative management or compared with other available therapies [3,8].

Because recent studies demonstrate that LVOT obstruction is associated with a worsened prognosis [13,14] and because there are different treatment options for obstructive HCM, it is important to evaluate the risks and benefits of myectomy, especially in its impact on survival. In this article we review the clinical course of

* Corresponding author. Division of Cardiology, Toronto General Hospital, University of Toronto, 200 Elizabeth Street, 4N 504, Toronto, ON M5G 2C4, Canada.
E-mail address: anna.woo@uhn.on.ca (A. Woo).

obstructive HCM and the effects of the presence of obstruction on the prognosis of HCM. The early and long-term results of surgery are outlined. We examine the outcomes of obstructive HCM in patients who undergo surgical versus conservative therapy. Finally, we review the results of the various other therapies available for the management of obstructive HCM.

Natural history and clinical course of obstructive hypertrophic cardiomyopathy

Classic studies on the clinical and hemodynamic features of HCM were performed at the National Institute of Health in the 1960s [6,15]. The original cohort of patients consisted of 64 patients who had a diagnosis of HCM, including 58 patients (91%) who had LVOT obstruction. No correlation was found between patients' symptoms and the magnitude of the LVOT gradient. There were 6 disease-related deaths, including 2 patients who died suddenly. The peak systolic pressure gradient of these 6 patients varied widely. The subsequent cohort consisted of 126 patients who had HCM, including 119 patients (94%) who had the obstructive form of HCM [15]. During the follow-up period, there were 10 cardiac deaths, including 6 SCDs, among the conservatively treated patients. The average resting LVOT gradient of the patients who died suddenly was lower than the LVOT gradient in the other 120 patients (23 versus 56 mm Hg, respectively [$P < .01$]). Furthermore, only 3 of the patients who died of a cardiac cause had an LVOT gradient greater than 30 mm Hg. Because most of the patients who died suddenly had no or mild obstruction, the authors suggested that mortality from HCM was not necessarily related to the presence of LVOT obstruction [15].

Subsequent studies from the 1970s demonstrated that the prognosis of obstructive HCM was unfavorable, with a high disease-related mortality rate and variable response to treatment [16–18]. The clinical course of 60 patients who had obstructive HCM (evaluated between 1958 and 1969) was reviewed by Adelman and colleagues [16]. The mortality rate was 14% (4 cardiac deaths) in 28 patients who had obstructive HCM who received either propranolol or no treatment. At the time of death these 4 patients were, on average, 40 years old. Another study of 119 patients who had obstructive HCM reported 30 deaths (25% mortality rate) during a mean follow-up of

4.6 years [17]. These findings were extended in a retrospective multicenter study from four centers, which assessed the clinical outcomes of 190 patients who had obstructive HCM [18]. Patients in this cohort were required to have a minimum of 1 year of follow-up and the mean follow-up time was 5 years. Management was divided into no specific treatment (31 patients), propranolol therapy (101 patients), or surgery (58 patients). The overall mortality rate was 26%. The cardiac mortality rate was 23% in the patients who received no specific treatment, 19% in the patients who were on propranolol, and 33% (including an operative mortality rate of 26%) in the patients who underwent surgery. In the 132 patients who were treated conservatively (ie, propranolol or no specific therapy) the cardiac mortality rate was 20% [18].

In the last 2 decades, however, multiple long-term studies have shown that the overall prognosis of HCM is more benign than described in earlier studies [3,4,19–21]. These study populations were largely derived from regional cohorts instead of tertiary care referral centers, and most patients included in these cohorts had nonobstructive HCM. The proportion of patients who had LVOT obstruction was 20% in the study by Spirito and colleagues [19] and by Cecchi and colleagues [20] and was 31% in the study by Maron and colleagues [21]. The annual cardiac mortality rate was 0.6% in the study by Cecchi and colleagues [20] and 1.3% in the study by Maron and colleagues [21]. In the latter study, the mortality of the 234 adult patients who had HCM was no greater than the expected mortality in the United States general population [21].

Long-term risks of left ventricular outflow tract obstruction in patients who have hypertrophic cardiomyopathy

The long-term impact of LVOT obstruction on the clinical outcome of HCM was analyzed in a large multicenter study of 1101 patients (273 [25%] who had a resting LVOT gradient ≥ 30 mm Hg), 828 [75%] who did not have obstruction) initially evaluated between 1983 and 2001 and followed for 6.3 ± 6.2 years [13]. Patients who had obstructive HCM had an increased risk for total mortality, HCM-related mortality, and SCD (Fig. 1). The probability of these endpoints was a relative risk of 2.0 (95% CI, 1.4–2.7, $P < .001$) for total mortality, a relative risk of 2.0 (95% CI, 1.3–3.0, $P = .001$) for HCM-related mortality,

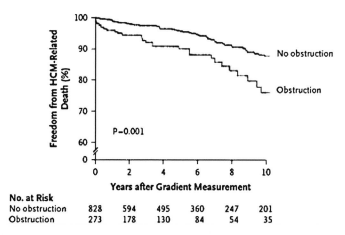

Fig. 1. Probability of HCM-related death among 273 patients who had a resting left ventricular outflow gradient of at least 30 mm Hg and 828 patients who did not have obstruction at entry. (*Reproduced from* Maron MS, Olivotto I, Betocchi S, et al. Effect of left ventricular outflow tract obstruction on clinical outcome in hypertrophic cardiomyopathy. N Engl J Med 2003;348:299; with permission. Copyright © 2003 Massachusetts Medical Society. All rights reserved.)

and a relative risk of 2.1 (95% CI, 1.1–3.7, P = .02) for SCD. The presence of LVOT obstruction was independently associated with HCM-related mortality (relative risk, 1.6; P = .02) and SCD (relative risk, 1.9; P = .01) on age-adjusted multivariable analysis. These findings were corroborated in another study of 917 patients who had HCM (288 [31%] with obstruction, 629 [69%] without obstruction) referred to St George's Hospital (United Kingdom) between 1988 and 2002 [14]. The 5-year survival from all-cause mortality/cardiac transplantation (86.5% [95% CI, 81.7–91.2] versus 90.1% [95% CI, 87.3–92.8], P = .006) and from SCD/appropriate implantable cardioverter-defibrillator [ICD] discharge (91.4% [95% CI, 87.4–95.3] versus 95.7 [95% CI, 93.8–97.6], P = .0004) was significantly lower in patients who had obstructive versus nonobstructive HCM, respectively. The presence of LVOT obstruction was associated with a low positive predictive value for SCD (7% and 10%) and a high negative predictive value (95% and 96%) in both studies, however [13,14].

Early surgical experience in hypertrophic cardiomyopathy

Surgery was first described as a treatment for HCM by Cleland and colleagues [5]. Cleland successfully performed a transaortic septal myectomy on a symptomatic 42-year-old man. At the time there had been a limited number of reports in the literature of this condition [1,2]. During the

1960s several other investigators would also report their experience with surgery for obstructive HCM [22–27], and Cleland and colleagues published their results on additional series of patients [28,29]. Surgical exposure of the septum was obtained through the aorta [5,22,24,30], the left ventricle [23], left atrium [25], or right ventricle [26,27]. The surgical approach to obstructive HCM involved either performing a myotomy, which involved dividing the obstructing muscle ("dividers"), and/or performing a myectomy, which involved resecting the muscle ("resectors") [27]. The number of patients included in these surgical cohorts ranged from 1 to 26 patients. Although initial case series had no operative deaths [5,22–24], subsequent studies reported early operative mortality rates of 4% to 25% [26,29,31,32]. Surgery was being performed for this condition, despite the fact that the underlying mechanisms for LVOT obstruction (ie, systolic anterior motion of the mitral leaflet leading to contact of the leaflet with the hypertrophied interventricular septum and resultant obstruction to outflow during systole) had not yet been elucidated. When Morrow and Brockenbrough [22] described the septal myotomy procedure, they proposed that the myotomy interfered with the sphincter-like muscular "contraction ring" in the outflow tract. Although immediate operative results were encouraging, the mechanism of benefit from surgery was unclear [22,27,29]. Moreover, these early investigators also highlighted the issue that surgical intervention was essentially a palliative procedure that could improve symptoms but not cure the underlying condition [22,24,29].

Outcomes following septal myectomy

Outcomes of myectomy in the 1970s and 1980s

During the 1970s and 1980s there remained continued controversy regarding the management of obstructive HCM. Echocardiographic studies helped to determine the mechanisms responsible for LVOT obstruction [3,4,9]. Surgery evolved from the septal myotomy [22,24,30] to the myectomy, performed by way of a transaortic approach (Fig. 2) [3,12,33]. Surgical alternatives to subaortic resection, such as mitral valve replacement [34,35], were also proposed. In addition, medical therapy with beta-blockers had been introduced and was found to be effective in treating the symptoms of obstructive HCM [36–38]. The major concern regarding myectomy was the continued high early mortality rate following this procedure. Reported early mortality rates in publications from major centers during the 1970s ranged from 8% to 26% [18,39,40]. Furthermore, some investigators pointed out that the postoperative late annual

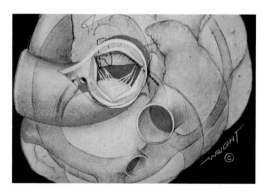

Fig. 2. Surgeon's view of the heart with the subaortic region visualized through an oblique aortotomy incision into the noncoronary sinus. Two longitudinal incisions are made in the basal septum. The incisions are connected proximally below the aortic valve and distally just beyond the level of mitral leaflet–septal contact. The myectomy specimen is excised to a depth that leaves 5 to 8 mm of residual septal wall thickness. Given the limited exposure to the ventricular septum, myectomy should be performed with intraoperative transesophageal echocardiographic guidance. (*From* Williams WG, Wigle ED, Rakowski H. Results of surgery for hypertrophic obstructive cardiomyopathy. Circulation 1987;76(Suppl V):V106; with permission.)

mortality rate in the largest series was 3.5% per year [40], which was comparable to the natural history of this condition [8]. Proponents of medical therapy argued that surgery therefore did not significantly improve the prognosis of patients who had obstructive HCM [7,8,41].

Contemporary outcomes of myectomy

Although publications from the 1980s and 1990s were still reporting early mortality rates of 5% to 8%, these results were largely because of the inclusion of cases from the 1960s and 1970s [12,42–44]. Multiple centers have demonstrated a significant decrease in the early postoperative mortality rates of more recent cohorts of patients undergoing myectomy (Table 1) [43–53]. This improvement in perioperative survival is likely because of such factors as increased understanding of the condition, the introduction of intraoperative echocardiography [11,54,55], and improved myocardial preservation techniques and postoperative care [12]. These contemporary studies of myectomy, largely involving cases performed since the late 1970s and performed at experienced surgical centers, have reported early mortality rates of 0% to 6%. Operative mortality for patients undergoing isolated myectomy has been lower than that of patients undergoing myectomy and a concomitant surgical procedure [46–53]. When the results from only the most recently published studies are considered (including the studies that have compared surgery to septal ethanol ablation), early mortality rates for isolated myectomy have generally been less than 1% (see Table 1; Table 2) [12,52,53]. The major limitation of myectomy at the present time is that surgical expertise is available only in a handful of selected tertiary referral centers [3,12].

Current surgical practice for treatment of obstructive hypertrophic cardiomyopathy

Pre- and postoperative transthoracic echocardiographic studies permit adequate visualization of the degree of septal hypertrophy and LVOT obstruction (Fig. 3). Myectomy is performed through an oblique aortotomy. This procedure requires intraoperative transesophageal echocardiographic guidance to assess the morphology of the hypertrophied septum, characterize the SAM and mitral regurgitation, determine the adequacy of the muscle resection, and rule out any significant complications [11]. Two longitudinal incisions are made in the basal septum. The incisions are

Table 1
Studies of early and long-term results of myectomy from experienced centers

Authors/year	Time period	Patients (N)	Early mortality (all cases) (%)	Early mortality (isolated myectomy) (%)	Mean follow-up time (y)	Survival at 5 y (%)	Survival at 10 y (%)
Cohn et al 1992 [46]	1972–1991	31	0	0	6.5	100	86
Schulte et al 1993 [44]	1963–1991	364	4.9[a]	2.9[b]	8.2	—	88
Ten Berg et al 1994 [47]	1977–1992	38	0	0	6.8	100	—
Heric et al 1995 [48]	1975–1993	178	6.2	4	3.7	86	70
Schoendube et al 1995 [49]	1979–1992	58	1.7	—	7.0	—	86
Robbins and Stinson 1996 [50]	1972–1994	158	3.2	2.3	6.1	85	72
Schoenbeck et al 1998 [51]	1965–1995	110	3.6	—	11.7	93	80
Woo et al 2005 [52]	1978–2002	338	1.5	0.8	7.7	95	83
Ommen et al 2005 [53]	1983–2001	289[c]	—	0.8	6.2	96	83

[a] 3.0% between years 1981 to 1990.
[b] 1.3% between years 1981 to 1990.
[c] Surgical cohort only included patients undergoing isolated myectomy.

connected proximally below the aortic valve and distally just beyond the level of mitral leaflet–septal contact. The resection may be extended more distally to the midventricular level (at the base of the papillary muscles) [3,12]. The length of the septal myectomy ranges from 35 to 50 mm, the width ranges from 20 to 35 mm (wider toward the apex than at the subaortic region), and the depth of the resection is aimed at leaving 8 to 10 mm of residual thickness at the site of the myectomy [52]. Concomitant surgical procedures are performed if necessary. At our institution, 26% of the 338 patients who underwent myectomy in our study required an additional surgical procedure: coronary artery

Table 2
Studies comparing left ventricular outflow tract gradients following septal ethanol ablation and myectomy

Study	No. of patients		Early deaths (%)		Resting LVOTG with SEA (mm Hg)		Resting LVOTG with myectomy (mm Hg)		Follow-up time
	SEA	Myectomy	SEA	Myectomy	Pre	Post	Pre	Post	
Qin et al 2001 [71]	25	26	0 (0%)	0 (0%)	64 ± 39	24 ± 19[a]	62 ± 43	11 ± 6[a]	3 months
Nagueh et al 2001 [70]	41	41	1 (2.4%)	0 (0%)	76 ± 23	8 ± 15	78 ± 30	4 ± 7	1 year
Firoozi et al 2002 [72]	20	24	1 (5%)	1 (4.2%)	91 ± 18	21 ± 12	83 ± 23	17 ± 12	28 months (SEA); 46 months (myectomy)
Ralph-Edwards et al 2005 [73]	54	48	1 (1.9%)	0 (0%)	74 ± 36	15[a]	64 ± 27	5[a]	1.8 years (SEA); 2.3 years (myectomy)
Van der Lee et al 2005 [74]	43	29	2 (4.7%)	0 (0%)	101 ± 34	23 ± 19	100 ± 20	17 ± 14	1 year

Abbreviations: LVOTG, left ventricular outflow tract gradient; SEA, septal ethanol ablation.
[a] $P < .01$ for resting LVOTG gradient post SEA versus myectomy.

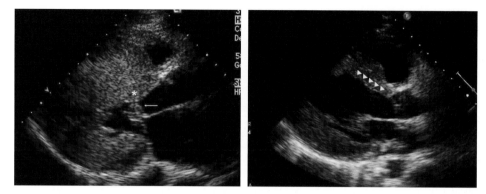

Fig. 3. Transthoracic two-dimensional echocardiographic studies in a 20-year-old man before (*left*) and after (*right*) transaortic septal myectomy. (*Left*) Parasternal long axis view of this patient, who presented with progressive class III symptoms of dyspnea, angina, and presyncope. The echocardiogram demonstrated massive septal hypertrophy (maximal septal thickness of 30 mm), near cavity obliteration in systole, severe systolic anterior motion of the anterior mitral leaflet (*arrow*), contact of the anterior mitral leaflet with the septum (*asterisk*), and a resting left ventricular outflow tract gradient of 100 mm Hg. (*Right*) Parasternal long axis view following surgery in the same patient. The echocardiogram now shows a widened left ventricular outflow tract because of the extensive resection of the proximal portion of the ventricular septum (*arrowheads*). There is no SAM and no detectable gradient in the left ventricular outflow tract.

bypass grafting (13%), unroofing of a coronary artery (7%), mitral valve repair or replacement (4%), aortic valve repair or replacement (2%), or right ventricular myectomy (2%) [52].

Does myectomy lower the risk for sudden death?

Although there was general agreement that surgery was effective in improving symptoms and relieving LVOT obstruction, it remained controversial whether surgery had an impact on the risk for SCD, the most devastating complication of HCM. Morrow and colleagues [56] argued that surgery and relief of the LVOT obstruction were effective in preventing SCD in survivors of cardiac arrest. They reported on a series of nine patients who had obstructive HCM who underwent myotomy and myectomy following a documented out-of-hospital cardiac arrest (caused by underlying ventricular fibrillation or ventricular tachycardia). The primary indication for surgery for these patients was the cardiac arrest and not significant exercise intolerance. In this study there was one early postoperative death and one late postoperative death (at 9 months following surgery). The latter patient was the only patient who did not have effective relief of his LVOT gradient following surgery. The surviving patients had no significant residual resting LVOT obstruction and remained free of a second cardiac arrest during postoperative follow-up. The authors postulated that the abolition of the LVOT gradient and the

reduction in left ventricular systolic pressure lessened ventricular electrical instability, decreased the recurrence rate of serious arrhythmias, and provided additional protection against the risk for SCD [56]. Other investigators have argued, however, that the low recurrence rate of cardiac arrest in these patients could be attributed to the use of antiarrhythmic medications during the postoperative follow-up period [8].

Studies of surgery versus conservative therapy in obstructive hypertrophic cardiomyopathy

There have been few studies that have directly compared survival in surgically treated versus conservatively treated patients who had HCM. Data from the 1970s had implied that surgery may have an impact on the SCD rate in patients who had obstructive HCM. In the multicenter nonrandomized study by Shah and colleagues [18], the outcomes of 190 patients who had obstructive HCM were assessed. Patients were treated conservatively (132 patients) or underwent surgery (58 patients). The mean follow-up time was 5 years. The cardiac mortality rate was 23% in the patients who were on no treatment, 19% in the patients on propranolol, and 33% in the patients who underwent surgery. The SCD rate was 16% in the untreated group and 18% in the propranolol group (SCD rate was 17% when these two groups were considered together). In the surgically treated group, there were 15 operative deaths (26%). There were 3 subsequent SCDs among the 43 survivors of surgery (7% rate of SCD among the survivors of surgery). This SCD rate in patients following surgery was balanced against the high operative mortality rate. Although the authors of this study suggested that surgery might be protective against the risk for SCD, they emphasized the obvious importance of having an acceptably low operative mortality rate in order to be able to recommend this treatment for patients who have symptomatic obstructive HCM [18].

Medical and surgical strategies for the treatment of obstructive HCM were compared in a cohort of patients evaluated at the same surgical center [57]. This was a nonrandomized single-center study of 112 patients who had HCM who were referred for myectomy (63 patients operated on between 1965 and 1980) or nonsurgical treatment (49 patients). Although the two groups were similar in age, the patients who underwent myectomy had more symptoms and a higher LVOT gradient (77 versus 30 mm Hg, surgical versus nonsurgical, respectively). The operative mortality rate was 1.6%. Ten-year survival was 80% in the surgical group and 71% in the nonsurgical group, although this difference was not statistically significant [57].

In a larger follow-up study to the work by Rothlin and colleagues [57], investigators from the same institution reported on the survival of

medically versus surgically treated patients [58]. This was a retrospective single-center study that analyzed 139 patients who had HCM referred since 1961. Treatment assignment to these two groups was not randomized and, in fact, patients were systematically allocated to medical therapy (60 patients) or surgical therapy (79 patients) based on the following institutional policy: (1) patients were treated medically if they had no or mild LVOT obstruction (< 50 mm Hg), or (2) patients were treated surgically if they had significant obstruction (defined as a resting LVOT gradient > 50 mm Hg or a provocable LVOT gradient > 100 mm Hg) or symptoms unresponsive to medications. The disease severity in the two treatment groups was therefore fundamentally different. The baseline resting LVOT gradient was 17 ± 21 mm Hg in the conservative group and 70 ± 33 mm Hg in the surgical group ($P < .05$). The early postoperative mortality rate was 1.3%. Despite having milder baseline LVOT obstruction, 10-year cumulative survival was significantly lower in the conservative group compared with the surgical group (68% versus 84%, $P < .05$) (Fig. 4) [58].

The results of the above studies did not resolve the issue of whether there were long-term survival benefits with myectomy, when performed with minimal perioperative mortality and morbidity, as compared with medical therapy in patients who had similar degrees of LVOT obstruction. Survival

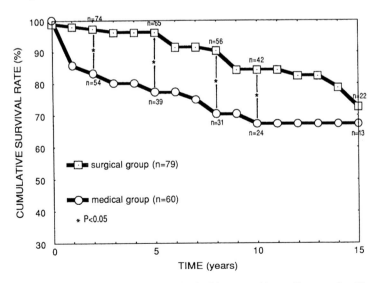

Fig. 4. Cumulative survival rates of the 139 patients who had hypertrophic cardiomyopathy. The surgically treated group had higher 2-, 5-, 8-, and 10-year survival rates than the medically treated group. (*Reproduced from* Seiler C, Hess OM, Schoenbeck M, et al. Long-term follow-up of medical versus surgical therapy for hypertrophic cardiomyopathy: a retrospective study. J Am Coll Cardiol 1991;17:638; with permission. Copyright © 1991, American College of Cardiology Foundation.)

in surgically versus nonsurgically treated patients who had obstructive HCM was assessed in a large retrospective observational study by Ommen and colleagues [53]. The survival of surgically treated patients was also compared with patients who had nonobstructive HCM and to the age- and gender-matched United States general population. This study consisted of 1337 patients who had HCM (517 patients who had obstructive HCM, 820 patients who had nonobstructive HCM) evaluated from 1983 to 2001. Three cohorts of patients were assembled: (1) patients who had obstructive HCM who underwent myectomy (289 patients undergoing isolated myectomy at the Mayo Clinic, Rochester, Minnesota), (2) nonoperated patients who had obstructive HCM (228 patients), and (3) patients who had nonobstructive HCM (820 patients). The latter two groups (1048 patients) were composed of patients evaluated at one of three HCM centers in the United States or Italy (and selected data were previously published) [13]. Mean follow-up duration was 6 ± 6 years. This study differed importantly from earlier studies that attempted to compare surgical and conservative therapies: (1) the patients in the different treatment groups (surgical and nonsurgical therapy) were managed at completely different institutions (surgical cases were all from the Mayo Clinic and nonsurgical cases were all from the other three institutions) and (2) the patients who had obstructive HCM in the surgical and nonsurgical therapy groups

had similar initial resting LVOT gradients (67 ± 41 versus 68 ± 31 mm Hg, respectively, P = .9). The surgical group was younger (45 ± 19 versus 50 ± 22 years, surgical versus nonsurgical, respectively, P < .01) and reported greater symptoms (89% versus 15% with class III or IV symptoms, respectively, P < .01) than the nonsurgical group.

Among the 517 patients who had obstructive HCM, overall survival was superior in the myectomy patients compared with the nonoperated patients (overall survival was 98%, 96%, and 83% versus 90%, 79%, and 61% at 1, 5, and 10 years, respectively, P < .001). The operative mortality rate was 0.8% in this cohort. Survival free from HCM-related death was also better in the myectomy patients compared with the nonoperated obstructive HCM patients (99%, 98%, and 95% versus 94%, 89%, and 73%, respectively, P < .001) (Fig. 5). Finally, the risk for SCD was lower in patients who underwent myectomy compared with nonoperated patients who had obstructive HCM (100%, 99%, and 99% versus 97%, 93%, and 89%, respectively, P = .003). On multivariable analysis, the only independent predictors of improved overall survival were myectomy (hazard ratio [HR] = 0.43, P < .001) and younger age at study entry (HR = 0.97 per year decrement of age, P < .001).

When survival was compared between the myectomy group and the patients who had

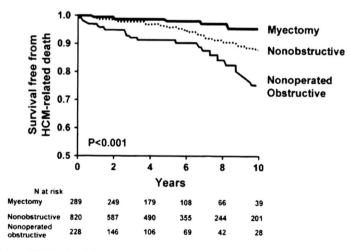

Fig. 5. Survival free from HCM-related death among patients in three subgroups: surgical myectomy (n = 289), nonoperated with obstruction (n = 228), and nonobstructive (n = 820). Overall log-rank, P < .001; myectomy versus nonoperated obstructive HCM, P < .001; myectomy versus nonobstructive HCM, P = .01. (*Reproduced from* Ommen SR, Maron BJ, Olivotto I, et al. Long-term effects of surgical septal myectomy on survival in patients with obstructive hypertrophic cardiomyopathy. J Am Coll Cardiol 2005;46:473; with permission. Copyright © 2005, American College of Cardiology Foundation.)

nonobstructive HCM, no statistically significant difference in overall survival was observed (98%, 96%, and 83% versus 98%, 95%, and 87%, respectively, $P = .8$). HCM-related survival was superior in the patients who underwent myectomy compared with the patients who had nonobstructive HCM (99%, 98%, and 95% versus 98%, 96%, and 91%, respectively, $P = .01$). Finally, there was no difference in overall survival between the surgically treated patients and the general population (98%, 96%, and 83% versus 98%, 95%, and 88%, respectively, $P = .2$). The authors therefore suggested that myectomy may allow patients to achieve normal or near-normal longevity.

In addition, a secondary analysis was performed in this study to assess the survival of young patients who had obstructive HCM (defined as age ≤ 45 years old at study entry) to reduce potentially confounding age-related comorbidities. Patients who underwent myectomy continued to demonstrate improved survival compared with nonoperated patients who had obstructive HCM (overall survival HR = 0.28, $P < .001$; HCM-related survival HR = 0.25; $P = .004$) in this younger subgroup. Overall survival was 99%, 98%, and 92% versus 92%, 88%, and 75%, at 1, 5, and 10 years, respectively ($P = .006$) [53].

There were significant limitations to this study, however. The most important shortcoming was that there were significant referral and selection biases in the compilation of the patient cohorts: all of the surgical subjects were referred to a tertiary referral center (Mayo Clinic) with an established expertise in myectomy, whereas the two nonsurgical groups were drawn from the other three centers [59]. Moreover, because patients who had obstructive HCM and major comorbidities (unrelated to the HCM itself) are more likely to not be offered surgery, patients who undergo surgery tend to be healthier. Nonsurgically treated patients may therefore have inherent characteristics that contribute to a worsened prognosis independent of the treatment strategy (surgery or conservative therapy) [59].

Determinants of long-term survival following myectomy

Because multiple options are available for the treatment of obstructive HCM, it is important to define which patients would benefit most from surgical intervention. We studied the clinical and echocardiographic predictors of long-term survival in patients following myectomy. Our study cohort consisted of 338 consecutive adult patients (mean age of 47 ± 14 years, septal thickness of 22 ± 5 mm, resting LVOT gradient of 66 ± 32 mm Hg, LA diameter of 46 ± 7 mm at surgery) operated on at our institution, Toronto General Hospital, between 1978 and 2002 [52]. The majority of the study subjects, 249 patients (74%), underwent an isolated myectomy procedure and 89 patients (26%) underwent myectomy and an additional cardiac surgical procedure.

Early postoperative mortality

The early postoperative mortality rate was 1.5%. There were five deaths in total: four deaths occurred between 1978 and 1992, and one death occurred between 1993 and 2002. There have been no early postoperative deaths in the last 145 consecutive cases included in our study cohort. The mortality rate was 0.8% (two deaths) among the 249 patients who underwent isolated myectomy and 3.4% (three deaths) among the 89 patients who had a concomitant surgical procedure ($P = .09$). Our early postoperative results are similar to the 0.8% operative mortality rate of isolated myectomy reported by Ommen and colleagues [53].

Long-term survival following myectomy

During a mean follow-up time of 7.7 ± 5.7 years (range, 1 day to 25.8 years), there was a total of 56 deaths (17%). Overall survival was 98% $\pm$ 1% at 1 year, 95% $\pm$ 1% at 5 years, and 83% $\pm$ 3% at 10 years following myectomy. The survival of patients following myectomy was compared with the survival of age- and gender-matched controls (subjects who did not have a history of coronary artery disease) from the population of Ontario, Canada. The control population had a survival of 97% $\pm$ 0.2% at 1 year, 96% $\pm$ 0.2% at 5 years, and 94% $\pm$ 0.4% at 10 years. Cardiovascular deaths accounted for 77% of all the deaths in our study population. Cardiovascular survival was 98% $\pm$ 1% at 1 year, 96% $\pm$ 1% at 5 years, and 87% $\pm$ 3% at 10 years. On multivariable analysis we found five predictors of overall mortality: (1) age 50 years or more at surgery (HR 2.8, 95% CI, 1.5–5.1, $P = .001$), (2) female gender (HR 2.5, 95% CI, 1.5–4.3, $P = .0009$), (3) history of preoperative AF (HR 2.2, 95% CI, 1.2–4.0, $P = .008$), (4) concomitant CABG (HR 3.7, 95% CI, 1.7–8.2, $P = .001$), and (5) preoperative LA diameter 46 mm or greater (HR 2.9, 95% CI, 1.6–5.4, $P = .0008$)

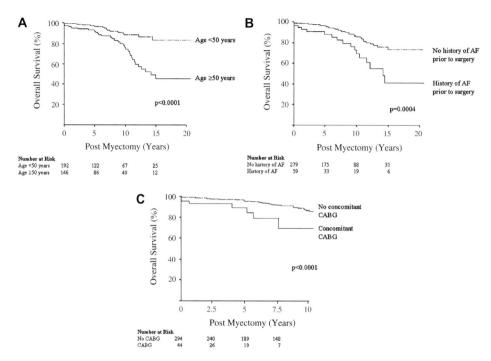

Fig. 6. Kaplan-Meier survival curves of overall postmyectomy survival stratified by (A) age (P < .0001), (B) history of preoperative atrial fibrillation (P = .0004), and (C) need for concomitant coronary artery bypass graft surgery (P < .0001). (*Reproduced from* Woo A, Williams WG, Choi R, et al. Clinical and echocardiographic determinants of long-term survival after surgical myectomy in obstructive hypertrophic cardiomyopathy. Circulation 2005;111:2037; with permission.)

(Fig. 6). These five variables were also found to be significant predictors of cardiovascular mortality and of late mortality (defined as total mortality excluding early postoperative mortality) [52].

Comparison of nonpharmacologic treatment strategies for obstructive hypertrophic cardiomyopathy

Dual chamber pacing versus myectomy

Initial studies of DDD atrioventricular pacing for the treatment of LVOT obstruction were promising [60,61]. Subsequent randomized crossover studies of DDD pacing (treatment arm) versus sham pacing (control arm) have shown an incomplete reduction in the LVOT gradient and no significant LV mass regression [62–64]. The perceived decline in symptoms following pacemaker implantation has been attributed, in part, to a placebo effect [62]. These findings were corroborated by a single-center nonrandomized study comparing DDD pacing and septal myectomy, which showed a significantly greater

improvement in symptoms, oxygen consumption, and the LVOT gradient in the patients who underwent surgery [65].

Septal ethanol ablation versus myectomy

SEA is an interventional technique that consists of the targeted infarction of the proximal septum by way of selective injection of ethanol into the septal perforator branch of the left anterior descending artery [66]. The localized infarction of the hypertrophied septum results in focal septal thinning, widening of the outflow tract, and relief of the LVOT obstruction [67]. The results of SEA are improved when it is guided by intraprocedural contrast echocardiographic guidance, which has become an essential part of the procedure [68,69]. Although there is the perception that SEA is relatively easy to perform, it is challenging from technical and echocardiographic standpoints and requires thorough understanding of HCM and the pathophysiology of LVOT obstruction [69]. There have been five nonrandomized studies that have compared septal ethanol ablation (SEA) with myectomy [70–74]. No significant differences in cardiac mortality during early and midterm follow-up were identified. Early procedural morbidity was higher in patients undergoing SEA; these patients were more likely to develop atrioventricular block and require permanent pacing [70–73]. There were similar improvements in the functional class and in the resting LVOT gradients following both procedures (see Table 2) [70–74]. The greatest difference in the resting LVOT gradients between the two treatment groups occurred at 3 months after the procedure, when patients who underwent SEA had higher resting LVOT gradients [71]. The earlier improvement in the LVOT gradient following myectomy is attributable to the immediate relief of LVOT obstruction with the resection of subaortic muscle, whereas the effect on the gradient with SEA is more gradual [75,76]. The maximal reduction in the LVOT gradient generally occurs more than 1 year following SEA [75,76]. Furthermore, although the long-term benefits of myectomy have been well demonstrated, the long-term sequelae of SEA have yet to be determined. In particular, it remains unclear whether the ethanol-induced infarction results in an increase in ventricular arrhythmias during long-term follow-up [77,78]. Myectomy should definitely be performed instead of SEA in the following settings: the presence of coexistent conditions (eg, coronary artery disease, intrinsic mitral valve disease), massive septal hypertrophy, coronary anatomy not amenable to ethanol injection, or the requirement for an acute reduction in the LVOT gradient [12].

Summary

Much has been learned about HCM in the past five decades. It is now recognized that patients who have HCM do not have a uniformly poor prognosis. Our increased understanding of the mechanism of LVOT obstruction has permitted the development of multiple therapies to treat the LVOT gradient. Patients who have obstructive HCM and symptoms uncontrolled by pharmacotherapy are candidates for myectomy or septal ethanol ablation. It cannot be overstated that both procedures need to be performed at centers with technical, clinical, and echocardiographic expertise in the management of HCM.

Given the relatively low prevalence of drug-refractory symptomatic obstructive HCM, the requirement for extended follow-up, and the paucity of centers with sufficient experience in both procedures, no prospective randomized controlled trials comparing these two treatment strategies have been completed. Nevertheless, myectomy is an established procedure that definitely abolishes symptoms and LVOT obstruction and results in excellent long-term survival. Recent data confirm that perioperative mortality is acceptably low when performed at experienced centers, and perioperative morbidity is lower than that reported following septal ethanol ablation. There are no studies that have demonstrated that myectomy (or any other intervention to reduce the LVOT gradient) improves the survival of asymptomatic patients who have obstructive HCM. Several observational studies provide suggestive evidence that the overall prognosis of patients who have symptomatic obstructive HCM is improved following surgery, however. Myectomy should therefore remain the gold standard of therapy for the treatment of symptomatic LVOT obstruction in patients who have HCM.

References

[1] Brock R. Functional obstruction of the left ventricle (acquired aortic subvalvar stenosis). Guys Hosp Rep 1957;106:221–38.
[2] Teare D. Asymmetrical hypertrophy of the heart in young adults. Br Heart J 1958;20:1–8.
[3] Maron BJ, McKenna WJ, Danielson GK, et al. Task force on clinical expert consensus documents. American College of Cardiology; Committee for Practice Guidelines. European Society of Cardiology. American College of Cardiology/European Society of Cardiology clinical expert consensus document on hypertrophic cardiomyopathy. A report of the American College of Cardiology Foundation Task Force on Clinical Expert Consensus Documents and the European Society of Cardiology Committee for Practice Guidelines. J Am Coll Cardiol 2003;42:1687–713.
[4] Maron BJ. Hypertrophic cardiomyopathy: a systematic review. JAMA 2002;287:1308–20.
[5] Goodwin JF, Hollman A, Cleland WP, et al. Obstructive cardiomyopathy simulating aortic stenosis. Br Heart J 1960;22:403–14.
[6] Braunwald E, Lambrew CT, Rockoff SD, et al. Idiopathic hypertrophic subaortic stenosis: I. A description of the disease based on an analysis of 64 patients. Circulation 1964;30(Suppl 4):3–119.
[7] Goodwin JF. An appreciation of hypertrophic cardiomyopathy. Am J Med 1980;68:797–800.

[8] Canedo MI, Frank MJ. Therapy of hypertrophic cardiomyopathy: medical or surgical? Clinical and pathophysiologic considerations. Am J Cardiol 1981;48:383–7.

[9] Rakowski H, Sasson Z, Wigle ED. Echocardiographic and Doppler assessment of hypertrophic cardiomyopathy. J Am Soc Echocardiogr 1988;1: 31–47.

[10] Wigle ED, Adelman AG, Auger P, et al. Mitral regurgitation in muscular subaortic stenosis. Am J Cardiol 1969;24:698–706.

[11] Grigg LE, Wigle ED, Williams WG, et al. Transesophageal Doppler echocardiography in obstructive hypertrophic cardiomyopathy: clarification of pathophysiology and importance in intraoperative decision making. J Am Coll Cardiol 1992;20: 42–52.

[12] Maron BJ, Dearani JA, Ommen SR, et al. The case for surgery in obstructive hypertrophic cardiomyopathy. J Am Coll Cardiol 2004;44:2044–53.

[13] Maron MS, Olivotto I, Betocchi S, et al. Effect of left ventricular outflow tract obstruction on clinical outcome in hypertrophic cardiomyopathy. N Engl J Med 2003;348:295–303.

[14] Elliott PM, Gimeno JR, Tome MT, et al. Left ventricular outflow tract obstruction and sudden death risk in patients with hypertrophic cardiomyopathy. Eur Heart J 2006;27:1933–41.

[15] Frank S, Braunwald E. Idiopathic hypertrophic subaortic stenosis: clinical analysis of 126 patients with emphasis on the natural history. Circulation 1968; 37:759–88.

[16] Adelman AG, Wigle ED, Ranganathan N, et al. The clinical course in muscular subaortic stenosis: a retrospective and prospective study of 60 hemodynamically proved cases. Ann Intern Med 1972;77: 515–25.

[17] Hardarson T, De la Calzada CS, Curiel R, et al. Prognosis and mortality of hypertrophic obstructive cardiomyopathy. Lancet 1973;2:1462–7.

[18] Shah PM, Adelman AG, Wigle ED, et al. The natural (and unnatural) history of hypertrophic obstructive cardiomyopathy: a multicenter study. Circ Res 1974;34 and 35(Suppl II):II179–95.

[19] Spirito P, Chiarella F, Carratino L, et al. Clinical course and prognosis of hypertrophic cardiomyopathy in an outpatient population. N Engl J Med 1989; 320:749–55.

[20] Cecchi F, Olivotto I, Montereggi A, et al. Hypertrophic cardiomyopathy in Tuscany: clinical course and outcome in an unselected regional population. J Am Coll Cardiol 1995;26:1529–36.

[21] Maron BJ, Casey SA, Poliac LC, et al. Clinical course of hypertrophic cardiomyopathy in a regional United States cohort. JAMA 1999;281:650–5.

[22] Morrow AG, Brockenbrough EC. Surgical treatment of idiopathic hypertrophic subaortic stenosis: technic and hemodynamic results of subaortic ventriculomyotomy. Ann Surg 1961;154:181–9.

[23] Kirklin JW, Ellis FH Jr. Surgical relief of diffuse subvalvular aortic stenosis. Circulation 1961;24:739–42.

[24] Wigle ED, Chrysohou A, Bigelow WG. Results of ventriculomyotomy in muscular subaortic stenosis. Am J Cardiol 1963;11:572–86.

[25] Lillehei CW, Levy MJ. Transatrial exposure for correction of subaortic stenosis. J Am Med Assoc 1963; 1686:8–13.

[26] Cooley DA, Bloodwell RD, Hallman GL, et al. Surgical treatment of muscular subaortic stenosis: results from septectomy in twenty-six patients. Circulation 1967;35(Suppl 1):124–32.

[27] Wigle ED, Trimble AS, Adelman AG, et al. Surgery in muscular subaortic stenosis. Prog Cardiovasc Dis 1968;11:83–112.

[28] Cleland WP. The surgical management of obstructive cardiomyopathy. J Cardiovasc Surg 1963;4: 489–91.

[29] Bentall HH, Cleland WP, Oakley CM, et al. Surgical treatment and post-operative haemodynamic studies in hypertrophic obstructive cardiomyopathy. Br Heart J 1965;27:585–94.

[30] Morrow AG, Lambrew CT, Braunwald E. Idiopathic hypertrophic subaortic stenosis: II. Operative treatment and the results of pre- and postoperative hemodynamic evaluations. Circulation 1964; 30(Suppl IV):120–51.

[31] Bigelow WG, Trimble AS, Auger P, et al. The ventriculomyotomy operation for muscular subaortic stenosis. J Thorac Cardiovasc Surg 1966;52:514–24.

[32] Morrow AG, Fogarty TJ, Hannah H III, et al. Operative treatment in idiopathic hypertrophic subaortic stenosis: techniques and the results of preoperative and postoperative clinical and hemodynamic assessments. Circulation 1968;37:589–96.

[33] Morrow AG. Hypertrophic subaortic stenosis: operative methods utilized to relieve left ventricular outflow obstruction. J Thorac Cardiovasc Surg 1978;76: 423–30.

[34] Cooley DA, Leachman RD, Wukasch DC. Diffuse muscular subaortic stenosis: surgical treatment. Am J Cardiol 1973;31:1–6.

[35] McIntosh CL, Maron BJ. Current operative treatment of obstructive hypertrophic cardiomyopathy. Circulation 1988;78:487–95.

[36] Cohen LS, Braunwald E. Amelioration of angina pectoris in idiopathic hypertrophic subaortic stenosis with beta-adrenergic blockade. Circulation 1967;35:847–51.

[37] Flamm MD, Harrison DC, Hancock EW. Muscular subaortic stenosis: prevention of outflow obstruction with propranolol. Circulation 1968;38:848–58.

[38] Frank MJ, Abdulla AM, Canedo MI, et al. Long-term medical management of hypertrophic obstructive cardiomyopathy. Am J Cardiol 1978;42: 993–1001.

[39] Tajik AJ, Guiliani ER, Weidman WH, et al. Idiopathic hypertrophic subaortic stenosis: long-term surgical follow-up. Am J Cardiol 1974;34:815–22.

[40] Maron BJ, Merrill WH, Freier PA, et al. Long-term clinical course and symptomatic status of patients after operation for hypertrophic subaortic stenosis. Circulation 1978;57:1205–13.

[41] Goodwin JF, Oakley CM. Medical and surgical treatment of hypertrophic cardiomyopathy. Eur Heart J 1983;4(Suppl F):209–14.

[42] Maron BJ, Epstein SE, Morrow AG. Symptomatic status and prognosis of patients after operation for hypertrophic obstructive cardiomyopathy: efficacy of ventricular septal myotomy and myectomy. Eur Heart J 1983;4(Suppl F):175–85.

[43] Mohr R, Schaff HV, Danielson GK, et al. The outcome of surgical treatment of hypertrophic obstructive cardiomyopathy: experience over 15 years. J Thorac Cardiovasc Surg 1989;97:666–74.

[44] Schulte HD, Bircks WH, Loesse B, et al. Prognosis of patients with hypertrophic obstructive cardiomyopathy after transaortic myectomy. J Thorac Cardiovasc Surg 1993;106:709–17.

[45] Schulte HD, Borisov K, Gams E, et al. Management of symptomatic hypertrophic obstructive cardiomyopathy—long-term results after surgical therapy. Thorac Cardiovasc Surg 1999;47:213–8.

[46] Cohn LH, Trehan H, Collins JJ. Long-term follow-up of patients undergoing myotomy/myectomy for obstructive hypertrophic cardiomyopathy. Am J Cardiol 1992;70:657–60.

[47] Ten Berg JM, Suttorp MJ, Knaepan PJ, et al. Hypertrophic obstructive cardiomyopathy: initial results and long-term follow up after Morrow septal myectomy. Circulation 1994;90:1781–5.

[48] Heric B, Lytle BW, Millder DP, et al. Surgical management of hypertrophic obstructive cardiomyopathy. J Thorac Cardovasc Surg 1995;110:195–208.

[49] Schoendube FA, KLues HG, Reith S, et al. Long-term clinical and echocardiographic follow-up after surgical correction of hypertrophic obstructive cardiomyopathy with extended myectomy and reconstruction of the subvalvular mitral apparatus. Circulation 1995;92(Suppl 2):II122–7.

[50] Robbins RC, Stinson EB. Long-term results of left ventricular myotomy and myectomy for obstructive hypertrophic cardiomyopathy. J Thorac Cardiovasc Surg 1996;111:586–94.

[51] Schonbeck MH, Brunner-La Rocca HP, Vogt PR, et al. Long-term follow-up in hypertrophic obstructive cardiomyopathy after septal myectomy. Ann Thorac Surg 1998;65:1207–14.

[52] Woo A, Williams WG, Choi R, et al. Clinical and echocardiographic determinants of long-term survival after surgical myectomy in obstructive hypertrophic cardiomyopathy. Circulation 2005;111:2033–41.

[53] Ommen SR, Maron BJ, Olivotto I, et al. Long-term effects of surgical septal myectomy on survival in patients with obstructive hypertrophic cardiomyopathy. J Am Coll Cardiol 2005;46:470–6.

[54] Marwick TH, Stewart WJ, Lever HM, et al. Benefits of intraoperative echocardiography in the surgical management of hypertrophic cardiomyopathy. J Am Coll Cardiol 1992;20:1066–72.

[55] Ommen S, Park SH, Click RL, et al. Impact of intraoperative transesophageal echocardiography in the surgical management of hypertrophic cardiomyopathy. Am J Cardiol 2002;90:1022–4.

[56] Morrow AG, Koch JP, Maron BJ, et al. Left ventricular myotomy and myectomy in patients with obstructive hypertrophic cardiomyopathy and previous cardiac arrest. Am J Cardiol 1980;46:313–6.

[57] Rothlin ME, Gobet D, Haberer T, et al. Surgical treatment versus medical treatment in hypertrophic obstructive cardiomyopathy. Eur Heart J 1983;4(Suppl F):215–23.

[58] Seiler C, Hess OM, Schoenbeck M, et al. Long-term follow-up of medical versus surgical therapy for hypertrophic cardiomyopathy: a retrospective study. J Am Coll Cardiol 1991;17:634–42.

[59] Watkins H, McKenna WJ. The prognostic impact of septal myectomy in obstructive hypertrophic cardiomyopathy (Editorial Comment). J Am Coll Cardiol 2005;46:477–9.

[60] Fananapazir L, Cannon RO, Tripodi D, et al. Impact of dual-chamber permanent pacing in patients with obstructive hypertrophic cardiomyopathy with symptoms refractory to verapamil and β-adrenergic blocker therapy. Circulation 1992;85:2149–61.

[61] Fananapazir L, Epstein ND, Curiel RV, et al. Long-term results of dual-chamber (DDD) pacing in obstructive hypertrophic cardiomyopathy: evidence for progressive symptomatic and hemodynamic improvement and reduction of left ventricular hypertrophy. Circulation 1994;90:2731–42.

[62] Nishimura RA, Trusty JM, Hayes DL, et al. Dual-chamber pacing for patients with hypertrophic obstructive cardiomyopathy: a prospective randomized, double-blind cross-over study. J Am Coll Cardiol 1997;29:435–41.

[63] Kappenberger L, Linde C, Daubert C, et al. Pacing in hypertrophic obstructive cardiomyopathy. A randomized crossover study. Eur Heart J 1997;18:1249–56.

[64] Maron BJ, Nishimura RA, McKenna WJ, et al. Assessment of permanent dual-chamber pacing as a treatment for drug-refractory symptomatic patients with obstructive hypertrophic cardiomyopathy. A randomized, double-blind, cross-over study (M-PATHY). Circulation 1999;99:2927–33.

[65] Ommen SR, Nishimura RA, Squires RW, et al. Comparison of dual-chamber pacing versus septal myectomy for the treatment of patients with hypertrophic obstructive cardiomyopathy. J Am Coll Cardiol 1999;34:191–6.

[66] Sigwart U. Non-surgical myocardial reduction for hypertrophic obstructive cardiomyopathy. Lancet 1995;346:211–4.

[67] Flores-Ramirez R, Lakkis NM, Middleton KJ, et al. Echocardiographic insights into the mechanisms of relief of left ventricular outflow tract obstruction after nonsurgical septal reduction therapy in patients with hypertrophic obstructive cardiomyopathy. J Am Coll Cardiol 2001;37:208–14.

[68] Faber L, Seggewiss H, Gleichmann U. Percutaneous transluminal septal myocardial ablation in hypertrophic obstructive cardiomyopathy: results with respect to intraprocedural myocardial contrast echocardiography. Circulation 1998;98:2415–21.

[69] Monakier D, Woo A, Vannan MA, et al. Myocardial contrast echocardiography in chronic ischemic and nonischemic cardiomyopathies. Cardiol Clin 2004;22:269–82.

[70] Nagueh SF, Ommen SR, Lakkis NM, et al. Comparison of ethanol septal reduction therapy with surgical myectomy for the treatment of hypertrophic obstructive cardiomyopathy. J Am Coll Cardiol 2001;38:1701–6.

[71] Qin JX, Shiota T, Lever HM, et al. Outcome of patients with hypertrophic obstructive cardiomyopathy after percutaneous transluminal septal myocardial ablation and septal myectomy surgery. J Am Coll Cardiol 2001;38:1994–2000.

[72] Firoozi S, Elliott PM, Sharma S, et al. Septal myotomy-myectomy and transcoronary septal alcohol ablation in hypertrophic obstructive cardiomyopathy: a comparison of clinical, haemodynamic and exercise outcomes. Eur Heart J 2002;23:1617–24.

[73] Ralph-Edwards A, Woo A, McCrindle BW, et al. Hypertrophic obstructive cardiomyopathy: comparison of outcomes after myectomy or alcohol ablation adjusted by propensity score. J Thorac Cardiovasc Surg 2005;129:351–8.

[74] van der Lee C, ten Cate FJ, Geleijnse ML, et al. Percutaneous versus surgical treatment for patients with hypertrophic obstructive cardiomyopathy and enlarged anterior mitral valve leaflets. Circulation 2005;112:482–8.

[75] Seggewiss H, Faber L, Gleichmann U. Percutaneous transluminal septal ablation in hypertrophic obstructive cardiomyopathy. Thorac Cardiovasc Surg 1999;47:94–100.

[76] Fernandes VL, Nagueh SF, Wang W, et al. A prospective follow-up of alcohol septal ablation for symptomatic hypertrophic obstructive cardiomyopathy—the Baylor experience (1996–2002). Clin Cardiol 2005; 28:124–30.

[77] Wigle ED, Schwartz L, Woo A, et al. To ablate or to operate: that is the question! J Am Coll Cardiol 2001;38:1707–10.

[78] Knight CJ. Alcohol septal ablation for obstructive hypertrophic cardiomyopathy. Heart 2006;92: 1339–44.

ELSEVIER
SAUNDERS

Heart Failure Clin 3 (2007) 289–298

Valve Pathology in Heart Failure: Which Valves Can Be Fixed?

Martinus T. Spoor, MD[†], Steven F. Bolling, MD[*]

University of Michigan, Ann Arbor, MI, USA

Congestive heart failure (CHF) is a significant health burden whose impact is increasing around the world. As our population ages, medical advances that have extended our average life expectancy have also left more people living with chronic cardiac disease than ever before. In the United States alone, there are nearly 4.9 million suffering with heart failure with over 500,000 new patients diagnosed each year. Despite the significant improvements with medical management, patients who have CHF are repeatedly readmitted for inpatient care, and the vast majority will die within 3 years of diagnosis [1]. Heart transplantation has evolved to become the gold standard treatment for patients who have symptoms of severe congestive heart failure associated with end-stage heart disease. From an epidemiologic perspective, this treatment is "trivial" because less than 2800 patients in the United States are offered transplantation due to limitations of age, comorbid conditions, and donor availability. New surgical strategies to manage patients with severe end-stage heart disease have therefore evolved to cope with the donor shortage in heart transplantation and have included high-risk coronary artery revascularization [2–9], cardiomyoplasty [10,11], and high-risk valvular repair or replacement [12].

Surgical treatment of mitral valve disease

Geometric mitral reconstruction

Functional mitral regurgitation (MR) is a significant complication of end-stage cardiomyopathy and it may affect almost all patients who have heart failure as a preterminal or terminal event. Its presence in these patients is associated with progressive ventricular dilatation, an escalation of CHF symptomatology, and significant reductions in long-term survival estimated between only 6 and 24 months [2].

A firm understanding of the functional anatomy of the mitral valve is fundamental to the management of MR in heart failure. The mitral valve apparatus consists of the annulus, leaflets, chordae tendineae, and papillary muscles as well as the entire left ventricle (LV). Thus the maintenance of chordal, annular, and subvalvular continuity is essential for the preservation of mitral geometric relationships and overall ventricular function. As the ventricle fails, the progressive dilatation of the LV gives rise to MR, which begets more MR and further ventricular dilatation (Fig. 1). With postinfarction remodeling and lateral wall dysfunction, similar processes combine to result in ischemic mitral regurgitation. Left uncorrected, the end result of progressive MR and global ventricular remodeling is similar regardless of the etiology of cardiomyopathy. Incomplete leaflet coaptation, loss of the zone of coaptation, and regurgitation develop secondary to alterations in the annular–ventricular apparatus and ventricular geometry [3,4]. As the mitral valve annulus increases in size, an increasing amount of redundant mitral leaflet tissue, associated with a reduction of the size of the area of coaptation

[†] Formerly from the Section of Cardiac Surgery, University of Michigan, Ann Arbor, Michigan.

[*] Corresponding author. Section of Cardiac Surgery, University of Michigan, 1500 East Medical Center Drive, Ann Arbor, MI 48103.

E-mail address: sbolling@umich.edu (S.F. Bolling).

1551-7136/07/$ - see front matter © 2007 Elsevier Inc. All rights reserved.
doi:10.1016/j.hfc.2007.04.008

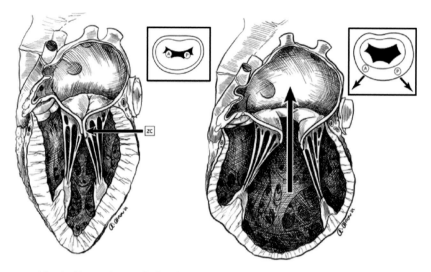

Fig. 1. Geometric ventricular changes with dilated myopathy, resulting in MR.

of the leaflet edges, becomes used in coverage of the surface area of the mitral valve orifice (Fig. 2). As more and more mitral leaflet tissue is used for coverage of the mitral valve orifice, a critical reduction in leaflet tissue available for coaptation is reached so that there is no longer an established zone of coaptation, and a central regurgitant jet of insufficiency begins to develop. This pathologic process has been referred to as "functional" mitral regurgitation. Thus, reconstruction of this geometric abnormality serves to not only restore valvular competency but also improve ventricular function [5–8].

Historically, the surgical approach to MR was mitral valve replacement, yet little was understood of the interdependence of ventricular function and annulus-papillary muscle continuity [9]. Consequently, patients who had low ejection fraction (EF) who underwent mitral valve replacement with removal of the subvalvular apparatus had prohibitively high mortality rates [10]. In an attempt to explain these outcomes, the concept of a beneficial "pop-off" effect of mitral regurgitation was conceived. This idea erroneously proposed that mitral incompetence provided a low-pressure relief during systolic ejection from the failing

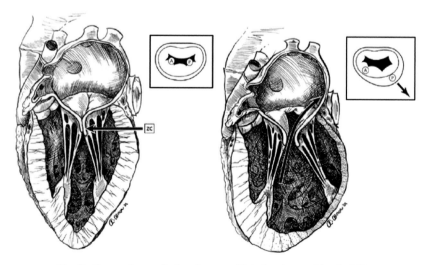

Fig. 2. Geometric ventricular changes with ischemia, resulting in MR.

ventricle, and that removal of this effect through mitral replacement was responsible for deterioration of ventricular function. Consequently, mitral valve replacement in patients who had heart failure was discouraged. More recent studies documenting the importance of maintaining subvalvular integrity to preserve postoperative LV function have led to surgical techniques that have been applicable to patients who had heart failure [11]. Accordingly, preservation of the mitral valve apparatus in mitral surgery has been demonstrated to enhance ventricular geometry, decrease wall stress, and improve systolic and diastolic function [12]. Therefore, maintenance of chordal, annular, and subvalvular continuity is essential for the preservation of optimal mitral geometry and overall ventricular function. Furthermore, preservation of the leaflet integrity as well as the dynamic function of the mitral apparatus with mitral repair has unmistakable functional benefits.

In treating patients who have heart failure, the most significant determinant of leaflet coaptation and MR is the diameter of the mitral valve annulus. The left-ventricular dimension is of less importance in functional MR, because the lengths of the chordae and papillary muscles are similar in myopathic hearts regardless of the presence of MR. Observations with medically managed patients who have severe heart failure and MR reveal that decreasing filling pressure and systemic vascular resistance lead to reductions in the dynamic MR associated with their heart failure [13]. This is attributed to a reduction in mitral orifice area relating to decreased LV volume and decreased annular distension. This complex relationship between mitral annular area and leaflet coaptation may thus explain why an undersized "valvular" repair may help a "ventricular" problem. This restoration of the mitral apparatus and ventricle forms the premise behind geometric mitral reconstruction for the treatment of heart failure.

At the University of Michigan, from 1992 to 2004, over 289 patients who had EF 30% or less received an undersized complete mitral annuloplasty ring as their mitral valve repair (MVR) procedure. Of these, 170 patients had a flexible complete ring while the remaining received a nonflexible undersized complete ring. In follow-up, 16 patients who had a flexible ring (9.4%) required a repeat procedure for significant recurrent geometric MR and CHF (10 replacements, 3 rerepairs, 3 transplants). The average time to reoperation was 2.4 years. In contrast, 119

patients who had an EF 30% or less received a MVR using an undersized nonflexible complete ring. Only 3 "nonflexible" patients required a repeat operation (1 required a MVR and 2 patients required a transplant). The time to reoperation was 4 years. There was a significant difference in reoperation rates for recurrent MR between the two groups ($P = .012$). There were no differences between groups in terms of age, ring size used, preoperative EF, LV size, MR grade or New York Heart Association (NYHA) class [14].

All patients were in NYHA class III or IV heart failure despite receiving maximal medical therapy. On immediate postoperative echocardiograms, the mean transmitral gradient has been 3 ± 1 mmHg (range 2–6 mm Hg). The overall operative mortality has been under 5%. There have been 27 late deaths: 12 from sudden ventricular arrhythmias, 9 from progression of CHF but without MR, 3 related to complications from other operative procedures, 2 that progressed to transplantation, and 1 suicide. The 1-, 2-, 3-, and 5-year actuarial survivals following geometric mitral reconstruction are 82%, 71%, 68%, and 57%, respectively.

At 24-month assessment, mean EF increased to 26%, and all patients were in NYHA class I or II. NYHA symptom scores were reduced from 3.2 ± 0.2 preoperatively to 1.8 ± 0.4 postoperatively. These improvements paralleled subjective functional improvements reported by all patients. By echocardiogram, there were marked improvements in regurgitant fraction, end-diastolic volume, cardiac output, and sphericity index. Although significant undersizing of the mitral annulus was employed to overcorrect for the zone of coaptation, no systolic anterior motion of the anterior leaflet or mitral stenosis was noted in these patients.

The technique of undersizing in mitral reconstruction avoids systolic anterior motion in these myopathic patients likely due to widening of the aorto-mitral angle in these hearts with increased LV size. Furthermore, acute remodeling of the base of the heart with this reparative technique may also re-establish the somewhat normal geometry and ellipsoid shape of the LV. As evidenced by the decreased sphericity index and LV volumes seen in these patients, the geometric restoration from mitral reconstruction not only effectively corrects MR but also achieves surgical unloading of the ventricle.

Many centers have reported similar consistent findings following geometric mitral reconstruction

[8,15–18]. With outcomes equating to transplant while avoiding immunosuppression, this straight-forward reparative operation performed in con-junction with medical management may be offered to all patients who have significant MR and cardiomyopathy as a first-line therapy.

The presence of mitral regurgitation is esti-mated to occur in 40% to 50% of patients who have heart failure. One recent study by Trichon estimated that in 30% of these patients, MR can be classified as either moderate or severe, which represents a large patient population given the high prevalence of heart failure [19]. The presence of increasing degrees of mitral regurgitation was associated with worsening prognosis, and even minor amounts of MR are associated with de-creased survival. Five-year survival is markedly worse as the degree of regurgitation increases [19].

Mitral stenosis

The overwhelming majority of patients pre-senting with hemodynamically significant mitral stenosis have preserved left-ventricular wall thick-ness, left-ventricular volume, and systolic and diastolic function in the absence of associated coronary artery disease [20,21]. Symptoms of CHF manifest from elevated pulmonary venous pressures as a result of obstruction to blood flow at the level of the mitral valve. Although unusual in this country in this current age, patients who have long-standing hemodynamically significant mitral stenosis may develop fixed and elevated pulmonary vascular resistance. As pulmonary vascular resistance rises, the pulmonary arteriolar bed becomes protected from sudden elevations in pressure associated with exertion, with the result that pulmonary edema does not occur, and pa-tients subsequently experience less symptoms of dyspnea. These patients, however, develop symp-toms of right-heart failure including peripheral coldness, cyanosis, hepatic enlargement and pul-sation, elevated jugular venous pressure, ascites, and peripheral edema. The risk of valve surgery in these patients is a consequence of pulmonary hypertension and right-heart dysfunction and not failure of the LV.

In some patients who have long-standing mitral stenosis, mild to modest degrees of poster-obasal regional wall contraction abnormalities may develop and may be attributed to a rigid mitral valve annulus and subvalvular apparatus [22]. However, significant impairment of left-ventricular function in association with hemodynamically significant mitral stenosis re-quiring operative treatment is an unusual finding but is present in a small proportion of patients. These patients tend to be elderly and have had long-standing mitral stenosis. These patients have been noted to have severe posterobasal seg-mental wall contraction abnormalities, anterolat-eral segmental contraction abnormalities, or diffuse hypokinesis [22–25]. The basis for the re-gional wall motion abnormalities may be related to diffuse scarring and retraction of the papillary muscles, and/or markedly decreased compliance of the LV. Chronic low cardiac output with signif-icantly decreased coronary flow reserves may contribute to diffuse hypokinesis and decreased left-ventricular compliance.

Surgical treatment of aortic valve disease

Aortic regurgitation

Aortic regurgitation may result from several causes including: (1) endocarditis; (2) inflamma-tory conditions such as rheumatic heart disease, syphilis, Takayasu's aortitis, or rheumatoid ar-thritis; (3) genetic disorders resulting in connective tissue abnormalities such as Marfan's or Ehlers-Danlos syndrome and their respective variants; (4) aortic dissection; or (5) congenital bicuspid aortic valve. These conditions elicit aortic regurgitation as a consequence of cusp perforation, annular dilation, cusp detachment, or leaflet scarring with ineffective leaflet coaptation.

Regurgitation from the aorta into the LV during diastole generates a volume *and* pressure overload to the LV. This elicits development of ec-centric hypertrophy of the LV, where left-ventric-ular wall thickness increases in proportion to the increase in ventricular diameter, such that the ra-tio between wall thickness and chamber radius re-mains normal. This adaptation in chronic aortic regurgitation permits the heart to maintain a good ejection fraction despite increases in left-ventricular end-diastolic volume. Patients who have chronic aortic regurgitation may remain well compensated and asymptomatic until late in their clinical course, despite a substantial volume load on the LV [26].

Bonow and colleagues [27–30] reported on the natural history of 77 asymptomatic patients who had normal left-ventricular ejection fraction at rest and severe aortic regurgitation (3+ to 4+ aor-tic regurgitation by ventriculography or pulse pressure > 70 mmHg). During a mean follow-up of 49 months, no patients died, and significantly, only 12 patients underwent aortic valve replacement (onset of symptoms [11 patients]; onset of left-ventricular dysfunction without symptoms [1 patient]). The percent of patients who did not require operation was $90 \pm 3\%$, $81 \pm 6\%$, and $75 \pm 7\%$, at 3, 5, and 7 years, respectively. Thus, in asymptomatic patients who had normal left-ventricular function, death is unusual, and less than 4% per year require aortic valve replacement because of the onset of symptoms or left-ventricular dysfunction. Subsequently Bonow reported on the natural history of 104 asymptomatic patients who had chronic severe aortic regurgitation and normal left-ventricular ejection fraction at rest. Of these 104 patients, $58\pm9\%$ remained asymptomatic with a normal ejection fraction at 11 years of follow-up (mean follow-up of 8 years) for an average attrition rate of less than 5% per year.

Thus, in the majority of patients who had asymptomatic severe chronic aortic regurgitation, the likelihood of the development of symptoms or onset of left-ventricular dysfunction is low, and the natural history is relatively benign. However, chronic volume overload in aortic regurgitation *eventually* leads to deterioration in left-ventricular systolic function. Ejection fraction and cardiac output eventually decline, and this is accompanied by an increase in the end-systolic volume. The primary basis for the onset of left-ventricular dysfunction remains controversial but has been postulated to be secondary to inadequate hypertrophy with afterload mismatch or primary myocardial dysfunction. Once symptoms of dyspnea, anginal, presyncope, or syncope develop, the average survival is only 3 to 5 years [26].

The decision to proceed with aortic valve surgery for chronic aortic regurgitation remains controversial and difficult because: (1) a large number of patients do well long-term without surgery; (2) patients undergoing aortic valve surgery after the onset of severe left-ventricular decompensation are less likely to improve symptomatically and are at increased risk of developing advanced heart failure within 5 years after surgery; and (3) asymptomatic patients who have aortic regurgitation may progress to irreversible left-ventricular dysfunction without perceptible symptomatic deterioration. Thus, asymptomatic or minimally symptomatic patients who have aortic regurgitation should be prospectively identified and offered aortic valve surgery before the point at which they develop irreversible left-ventricular dysfunction. Numerous studies have demonstrated that the overwhelming majority of symptomatic patients at risk of death from heart failure after operation have impaired systolic function *before* operation [31]. From these studies, several indices of the left-ventricular functional state have been identified that have important prognostic information in regard to the likelihood of requiring aortic valve replacement for chronic aortic regurgitation and the likelihood of successful short- and long-term outcome following operation. These indices have included ejection fraction at rest or in response to exercise, duration of left-ventricular dysfunction, fractional shortening, left-ventricular dimensions at end-systole and end-diastole, end-systolic and end-diastolic volume index, and end-diastolic radius to wall-thickness ratio. Thus, in symptomatic patients undergoing aortic valve surgery for aortic regurgitation, the postoperative survival, incidence of postoperative congestive heart failure, and likelihood of postoperative reversal of left-ventricular dilation can be predicted on the basis of preoperative left-ventricular systolic function, systolic size, and systolic wall stress.

These same variables also identify asymptomatic patients who have severe chronic aortic regurgitation and normal left-ventricular systolic function who are likely to require aortic valve replacement over the course of the next 4 years because of the development of symptoms or the onset of left-ventricular dysfunction [32]. Thus, when aortic valve replacement is delayed until the onset of either symptoms, left-ventricular dysfunction, or both, death before surgery is rare (limited to patients who have marked ventricular dilatation), and postoperative survival should be excellent with substantial improvement in left-ventricular dilatation and function, although there remains a poorly studied subset of patients who receive no survival benefit from the surgery and their long-term results are not as good.

However, although left-ventricular systolic dysfunction at rest is a sensitive means of detecting patients at risk, it is not specific, and improvement and even normalization of left-ventricular systolic function can occur in patients after operation despite severe depression of systolic function before operation. Left-ventricular function during exercise and exercise capacity has been used as additional indices to determine timing of operation for aortic insufficiency and provide prognostic information following surgery. Preserved exercise capacity before operation predicts improved survival after surgery and predicts postoperative reversibility of left-ventricular dysfunction. Further, abnormal ejection fraction during exercise may precede the onset of symptoms or the onset of resting left-ventricular dysfunction in many patients. However, left-ventricular dysfunction presented only during exercise should not be an indication for aortic valve surgery, but may identify a group of patients who need closer surveillance for other indices of left-ventricular dysfunction [33].

In summary, patients who have hemodynamically significant aortic regurgitation and symptoms of congestive heart failure (NYHA class III or IV), angina, or syncope should undergo aortic valve surgery. Asymptomatic or minimally symptomatic patients require serial assessments of left-ventricular size and function to determine the optimal timing of surgery. An exercise-tolerance test will ensure that patients are not masking symptoms by limiting activity. Asymptomatic patients who have left-ventricular enlargement are observed serially as long as left-ventricular function remains normal, but more recent studies are beginning to question this practice. Aortic valve surgery is recommended if left-ventricular function deteriorates by radionuclide or echocardiographic measures. Noninvasive studies, such as serial M-mode echocardiograms, are used to follow left-ventricular size and function and help predict which patients will likely have persistent postoperative left-ventricular dysfunction and a poor long-term prognosis. Asymptomatic patients, whose ventricular size is normal, are tested every year for deterioration in resting left-ventricular function (EF < 40%), increases in the end-systolic dimension to greater than 55 mm, or decreases in left-ventricular fractional shortening to less than 29%, understanding that waiting for symptomatic decompensation will compromise postoperative outcome. The rate of progression of left-ventricular dysfunction is also considered in the timing of aortic valve replacement, with rapid progression suggesting the need for earlier surgery. Shorter preoperative duration of left-ventricular dysfunction predicts the return of normal function postoperatively. Coronary angiography is performed in patients over the age of 45 years to assess the need for coronary artery revascularization.

Aortic stenosis

The two most common causes for hemodynamically significant aortic stenosis are congenital bicuspid aortic valve and degenerative calcific disease principally in elderly patients. The natural history of aortic stenosis is not completely understood given the advent of aortic valve replacement; but compared with aortic insufficiency, valvular aortic stenosis is characterized by a more malignant course in terms of survival following development of symptoms. The natural history of the disease reveals an average survival in patients who have significant aortic stenosis after the onset of heart failure symptoms was 1 to 2 years, 2 to 3 years following the onset of syncope, and 4 to 5 years following the onset of angina [34].

The transition from the asymptomatic to symptomatic stage of aortic stenosis has a profound effect on the natural history of this disease. The subsequent clinical course of hemodynamically significant aortic stenosis becomes malignant. Of patients who have severe, hemodynamically significant aortic stenosis (valve area ≤ 0.7 cm^2), 40% will develop symptoms within 1.5 to 2 years of diagnosis and most within 5 years [35]. The actuarial probability of remaining free of angina, syncope, or dyspnea is approximately 86% at 1 year and 62% at 2 years. Thus patients who have asymptomatic hemodynamically significant aortic stenosis are at significant risk for the development of cardiac events within 2 years of onset of symptoms. However, during the period they are asymptomatic, the risk of sudden death is low, approximately 1% per year [36].

The natural history of mild aortic stenosis (aortic valve area > 1.5 cm^2) is relatively benign. In a group of 142 patients followed to 10 years, aortic stenosis remained mild in 88% of patients and progressed to moderate aortic stenosis in 4%, while 8% of patients required aortic valve replacement [37]. At 20 years of follow-up, the aortic stenosis remained mild in 63% and progressed to moderate stenosis in 15%, while 22% of patients underwent aortic valve replacement or had severe aortic stenosis.

As has been the traditional surgical teaching, almost all patients who have aortic stenosis should be considered for aortic valve replacement. Conversely in aortic insufficiency in which deterioration of left-ventricular function develops early in the course of the disease and may reach a point of no return at which valve replacement can no longer produce clinical improvement, more caution is required. There are two reasons why such considerations do not apply to aortic stenosis. First, the great majority of patients has symptoms and undergoes operations when left-ventricular function is still normal or only mildly impaired. Second, when impaired left-ventricular function develops in aortic stenosis, the relief of pressure overload almost always restores normal function or at least produces considerable improvement with survival up to 55% at 10 years [38]. However, significant concomitant coronary artery disease can obviously obscure whether left-ventricular dysfunction is based on ischemic heart disease, valvular heart disease, or both.

Despite early symptomatic improvement following aortic valve replacement for aortic stenosis, there is a real and significant incidence of late return of congestive heart failure despite this early improvement [39]. The cause of this is likely multifactorial related to intrinsic and extrinsic patient factors. In patients who had obtained complete freedom from functional disability 1 year after aortic valve replacement, the recurrence of congestive heart failure noted at 10 years of follow-up is exclusively related to the starting point (ie, to advanced symptomatic disease before the operation). Almost two thirds of deaths occurring more than 12 years after aortic valve replacement, when the late excess mortality becomes prevalent, are caused by congestive heart failure. Thus the degree of myocardial fibrosis that occurs preoperatively as a result of aortic stenosis and correlates with the degree of hypertrophy may ultimately determine the long-term prognosis. Preoperative data is significantly predictive of left-ventricular performance more than 10 years after the operation, and impaired function in turn depended closely on residual hypertrophy. Preoperative factors predictive of late death following aortic valve replacement include peak-to-peak systolic gradient, cardiothoracic index, left-ventricular failure, prosthetic orifice diameter of 15 mm or less, age, ventricular ectopic beats, male gender, and anti-anginal/antiarrhythmic treatement [40].

In summary, the natural history of symptomatic, severe aortic stenosis is malignant, and aortic valve replacement is clearly indicated in the appropriate risk patient. The risk of sudden death in a *truly asymptomatic* patient who has severe aortic stenosis is not well defined but seems to approximate 1% to 2%. Thus aortic stenosis is not strictly indicated in the asymptomatic patient who has severe aortic stenosis to prevent sudden death. However, a substantial majority of these patients rapidly develop symptoms and thus aortic valve replacement becomes indicated. Asymptomatic patients who have severe aortic stenosis and impaired left-ventricular function should be advised to undergo aortic valve replacement. The course of patients who have symptomatic moderate aortic stenosis is clearly progressive, and significant mortality exists at 4 years after diagnosis. Thus, these patients require close follow-up and aortic valve replacement is indicated in the appropriate risk patient. The natural history of patients who have mild aortic stenosis or asymptomatic moderate aortic stenosis is relatively benign, and thus aortic valve replacement is not indicated. These patients, however, require good follow-up to identify progression of their disease.

Tricuspid valve disease

The association of significant tricuspid valve regurgitation in patients who have either aortic or mitral valve disease has often been noted in 10% to 35% of patients and results in a significant number of patients presenting for consideration of tricuspid valve surgery [41,42]. Persistent regurgitation following mitral valve surgery may resolve or improve, but in a subset of patients, it is associated with impaired cardiac output response and increasing symptoms [43]. One group showed that this was more likely to be the case in rheumatic patients with significant involvement of their mitral valve [44]. The well-known modified deVega annuloplasty is a straightforward surgical technique to apply to the tricuspid valve and does not significantly add to the length of the primary cardiac procedure. Some groups have advocated the routine use of a tricuspid annuloplasty procedure, while others favor a ring annuloplasty approach in terms of long-term durability of the repair [45,46].

Emerging valve surgery technologies

Emerging biomedical devices for heart failure

The Acorn Cardiac Support Device ([ACSD] Acorn Medical, Minneapolis, Minnesota) is a polyester mesh fabric that attempts to reduce ventricular wall stress by providing external support. The ACSD is placed around the ventricles from posterior to anterior, using stay sutures, as well as an anterior fabric seam for snug tailoring to the patient's heart.

Taking advantage of the girdling effect, the purpose of this device is to passively support the failing ventricles and prevent further dilatation. Preclinical data have shown decreased LV volumes and improvements in regional wall motion, EF, and other functional parameters without any evidence of constrictive physiology [47]. Histologic animal studies have also demonstrated decreased myocyte hypertrophy and interstitial fibrosis, as well as improvements in several biochemical markers of failure [48,49]. A phase I-II clinical trial has been completed to assess the safety and the early remodeling ability of the ACSD when used on patients who have heart failure with or without concomitant cardiac procedures. Although not currently approved by the FDA for general use, the device continues to remain under current investigation. Preliminary experience reveals that the ACSD is easily applied, and may even be performed without the necessity of cardiopulmonary bypass.

The Myocor Myosplint (Myocor Medical, St. Paul, Minnesota) is a second device developed to reduce ventricular wall stress by directly altering cardiac geometry. Working on the premise of optimizing the law of LaPlace, it involves the placement of transventricular tension bands through the right ventricle and LV walls that have the unique ability to be individually tightened to achieve a 20% reduction in wall stress. Preclinical animal data have shown improvements in end-diastolic volume, end-systolic volume, and EF. These experiments reveal the Myocor device becomes readily incorporated within a fibrous capsule that has been free of thrombus formation. A phase I clinical trial is under way to assess device safety in patients before cardiectomy at the time of transplant. Preliminary data reveal that the device can be readily deployed without harm to other cardiac structures. Further chronic studies are required to address the efficacy of this unique device.

The Geoform mitral valve annuloplasty ring (Edwards Lifesciences, Irvine, California) has a three-dimensional shape that attempts to combine the aforementioned principles of mitral valve repair and geometric remodeling of the LV into the next generation of mitral valve rings. This ring attempts to change and promote remodeling of the LV through alterations in the mitral valve apparatus. The basic anatomic problem in dilated LVs, whether from ischemia or not, is the tendency of the posterior mitral valve annulus to fall away from the annular plane, which further promotes increased mitral regurgitation and increased left-ventricular wall stress. Restoring the zone of coaptation of the mitral valve, using this ring, in the normal plane has two combined effects of correcting the mitral regurgitation and changing the shape of the LV. Based on the elegant and

pioneering efforts of Alfieri's group, the new geometry of the ventricle following this procedure has lower wall stress, which should promote further beneficial changes in the ventricle over time as the volume overload is relieved following correction of the mitral regurgitation [50]. The Geoform ring is currently approved for clinical use with multiple implants performed at several centers worldwide.

Percutaneous mitral valve repair

The Edwards Milano II mitral clip (Edwards Lifesciences, Irvine, California) and Evalve Mitraclip sytem (Evalve Inc, Menlo Park, California) uses a catheter-based approach to deliver a clip to the anterior and posterior mitral valve leaflets using the principles of mitral repair pioneered by Dr. Otavio Alfieri. Percutaneous catheters are introduced by way of the femoral vein and cross the atrial septum to enter the left atrium similar to a percutaneous mitral balloon annuloplasty approach. A catheter-based clip is then used to create a permanent coaptation point between the leading free edges of the anterior and posterior mitral leaflets. This technology is in the investigational stage with the Evalve clip currently being evaluated in the phase II EVEREST trial.

The Viacor percutaneous mitral annuloplasty system (Viacor Inc, Wilmington, Massachusetts), Edwards Viking percutaneous mitral annuloplasty system (Viking, Edwards Lifesciences Inc, Irvine, California), and Carillon mitral contour system (Cardiac Dimensions, Kirkland, Washington) all use an emerging technology approach to mitral annuloplasty using a catheter-based approach to the mitral valve. Using percutaneous catheters, a permanent nitinol strut is placed into the coronary sinus that wraps around the posterior annulus of the mitral valve and attempts to indirectly influence the action of the posterior mitral valve leaflet similar to a partial ring annuloplasty by reducing the anterior–posterior dimension of the mitral annulus. The devices are presently under investigational study and are not currently approved for routine use.

Percutaneous aortic valve replacement

Several groups are now attempting to develop techniques to replace the aortic valve using percutaneous approaches [51]. Most of these techniques have been attempted on patients not otherwise eligible for more conventional valve replacement using cardiopulmonary bypass, and the early results reflect this and have used catheter-based antegrade and retrograde approaches as well as transapical minithoractomy procedures [52]. Other groups are using the same concept to approach the pulmonary valve, which is the least likely valve to be addressed in the average adult population but whose importance will play an increasingly larger role in the rapidly expanding adult population that has congenital heart disease [53].

References

[1] Tavazzi L. Epidemiology of dilated cardiomyopathy: a still undetermined entity. Eur Heart J 1997; 18(1):4–6.

[2] Blondheim DS, Jacobs LE, Kotler MN, et al. Dilated cardiomyopathy with mitral regurgitation: decreased survival despite a low frequency of left ventricular thrombus. Am Heart J 1991;122(3 Pt 1): 763–71.

[3] Boltwood CM, Tei C, Wong M, et al. Quantitative echocardiography of the mitral complex in dilated cardiomyopathy: the mechanism of functional mitral regurgitation. Circulation 1983;68(3):498–508.

[4] Kono T, Sabbah HN, Rosman H, et al. Left ventricular shape is the primary determinant of functional mitral regurgitation in heart failure. J Am Coll Cardiol 1992;20(7):1594–8.

[5] Bach DS, Bolling SF. Improvement following correction of secondary mitral regurgitation in end-stage cardiomyopathy with mitral annuloplasty. Am J Cardiol 1996;78(8):966–9.

[6] Bolling SF, Deeb GM, Brunsting LA, et al. Early outcome of mitral valve reconstruction in patients with end-stage cardiomyopathy. J Thorac Cardiovasc Surg 1995;109(4):676–82 [discussion: 682–3].

[7] Bolling SF, Pagani FD, Deeb GM, et al. Intermediate-term outcome of mitral reconstruction in cardiomyopathy. J Thorac Cardiovasc Surg 1998;115(2): 381–6 [discussion: 387–88].

[8] Chen FY, Adams DH, Aranki SF, et al. Mitral valve repair in cardiomyopathy. Circulation 1998; 98(19 Suppl):II124–7.

[9] Pitarys CJ 2nd, Forman MB, Panayiotou H, et al. Long-term effects of excision of the mitral apparatus on global and regional ventricular function in humans. J Am Coll Cardiol 1990;15(3):557–63.

[10] Phillips HR, Levine FH, Carter JE, et al. Mitral valve replacement for isolated mitral regurgitation: analysis of clinical course and late postoperative left ventricular ejection fraction. Am J Cardiol 1981;48(4):647–54.

[11] David TE, Uden DE, Strauss HD. The importance of the mitral apparatus in left ventricular function after correction of mitral regurgitation. Circulation 1983;68(3 Pt 2):II76–82.

[12] Sarris GE, Cahill PD, Hansen DE, et al. Restoration of left ventricular systolic performance after reattachment of the mitral chordae tendineae. The importance of valvular-ventricular interaction. J Thorac Cardiovasc Surg 1988;95(6):969–79.

[13] Rosario LB, Stevenson LW, Solomon SD, et al. The mechanism of decrease in dynamic mitral regurgitation during heart failure treatment: importance of reduction in the regurgitant orifice size. J Am Coll Cardiol 1998;32(7):1819–24.

[14] Spoor MT, Geltz A, Bolling SF. Flexible versus nonflexible mitral valve rings for congestive heart failure: differential durability of repair. Circulation 2006;114(1 Suppl):I67–71.

[15] Bishay ES, McCarthy PM, Cosgrove DM, et al. Mitral valve surgery in patients with severe left ventricular dysfunction. Eur J Cardiothorac Surg 2000; 17(3):213–21.

[16] Bitran D, Merin O, Klutstein MW, et al. Mitral valve repair in severe ischemic cardiomyopathy. J Card Surg 2001;16(1):79–82.

[17] Calafiore AM, Gallina S, Di Mauro M, et al. Mitral valve procedure in dilated cardiomyopathy: repair or replacement? Ann thorac Surg 2001;71(4): 1146–52.

[18] Radovanovic N, Mihajlovic B, Selestiansky J, et al. Reductive annuloplasty of double orifices in patients with primary dilated cardiomyopathy. Ann Thorac Surg 2002;73(3):751–5.

[19] Trichon BH, Felker GM, Shaw LK, et al. Relation of frequency and severity of mitral regurgitation to survival among patients with left ventricular systolic dysfunction and heart failure. Am J Cardiol 2003; 91(5):538–43.

[20] Schuler G, Peterson KL, Johnson AD, et al. Serial noninvasive assessment of left ventricular hypertrophy and function after surgical correction of aortic regurgitation. Am J Cardiol 1979;44(4): 585–94.

[21] Halperin Z, Karasik A, Lewis BS, et al. Echocardiographic left ventricular function in mitral stenosis. Isr J Med Sci 1978;14(8):841–7.

[22] Heller SJ, Carleton RA. Abnormal left ventricular contraction in patients with mitral stenosis. Circulation 1970;42(6):1099–110.

[23] Bolen JL, Lopes MG, Harrison DC, et al. Analysis of left ventricular function in response to afterload changes in patients with mitral stenosis. Circulation 1975;52(5):894–900.

[24] Curry GC, Elliott LP, Ramsey HW. Quantitative left ventricular angiocardiographic findings in mitral stenosis. Detailed analysis of the anterolateral wall of the left ventricle. Am J Cardiol 1972;29(5):621–7.

[25] Holzer JA, Karliner JS, O'Rourke RA, et al. Quantitative angiographic analysis of the left ventricle in patients with isolated rheumatic mitral stenosis. Br Heart J 1973;35(5):497–502.

[26] Rapaport E. Natural history of aortic and mitral valve disease. Am J Cardiol 1975;35(2):221–7.

[27] Bonow RO, Dodd JT, Maron BJ, et al. Long-term serial changes in left ventricular function and reversal of ventricular dilatation after valve replacement for chronic aortic regurgitation. Circulation 1988; 78(5 Pt 1):1108–20.

[28] Bonow RO, Lakatos E, Maron BJ, et al. Serial long-term assessment of the natural history of asymptomatic patients with chronic aortic regurgitation and normal left ventricular systolic function. Circulation 1991;84(4):1625–35.

[29] Bonow RO, Picone AL, McIntosh CL, et al. Survival and functional results after valve replacement for aortic regurgitation from 1976 to 1983: impact of preoperative left ventricular function. Circulation 1985;72(6):1244–56.

[30] Bonow RO, Rosing DR, McIntosh CL, et al. The natural history of asymptomatic patients with aortic regurgitation and normal left ventricular function. Circulation 1983;68(3):509–17.

[31] Tamas E, Nylander E, Olin C. Are patients with isolated chronic aortic regurgitation operated in time? Analysis of survival data over a decade. Clin Cardiol 2005;28(7):329–32.

[32] Scognamiglio R, Negut C, Palisi M, et al. Long-term survival and functional results after aortic valve replacement in asymptomatic patients with chronic severe aortic regurgitation and left ventricular dysfunction. J Am Coll Cardiol 2005;45(7):1025–30.

[33] Supino PG, Borer JS, Herrold EM, et al. Prognostic impact of systolic hypertension on asymptomatic patients with chronic severe aortic regurgitation and initially normal left ventricular performance at rest. Am J Cardiol 2005;96(7):964–70.

[34] Ross J Jr, Braunwald E. Aortic stenosis. Circulation 1968;38(1 Suppl):61–7.

[35] Pellikka PA, Nishimura RA, Bailey KR, et al. The natural history of adults with asymptomatic, hemodynamically significant aortic stenosis. J Am Coll Cardiol 1990;15(5):1012–7.

[36] Pellikka PA, Sarano ME, Nishimura RA, et al. Outcome of 622 adults with asymptomatic, hemodynamically significant aortic stenosis during prolonged follow-up. Circulation 2005;111(24):3290–5.

[37] Horstkotte D, Loogen F. The natural history of aortic valve stenosis. Eur Heart J 1988;9(Suppl E):57–64.

[38] Chukwuemeka A, Rao V, Armstrong S, et al. Aortic valve replacement: a safe and durable option in patients with impaired left ventricular systolic function. Eur J Cardiothorac Surg 2006;29(2):133–8.

[39] Cohen G, David TE, Ivanov J, et al. The impact of age, coronary artery disease, and cardiac comorbidity on late survival after bioprosthetic aortic valve replacement. J Thorac Cardiovasc Surg 1999;117(2):273–84.

[40] Lund O. Preoperative risk evaluation and stratification of long-term survival after valve replacement for aortic stenosis. Reasons for earlier operative intervention. Circulation 1990;82(1):124–39.

[41] King RM, Schaff HV, Danielson GK, et al. Surgery for tricuspid regurgitation late after mitral valve replacement. Circulation 1984;70(3 Pt 2):I193–7.

[42] Barlow JB. Aspects of mitral and tricuspid regurgitation. J Cardiol 1991;25:3–33.

[43] Groves PH, Ikram S, Ingold U, et al. Tricuspid regurgitation following mitral valve replacement: an echocardiographic study. J heart Valve Dis 1993; 2(3):273–8.

[44] Lim E, Ali ZA, Barlow CW, et al. Determinants and assessment of regurgitation after mitral valve repair. J Thorac Cardiovasc Surg 2002;124(5):911–7.

[45] Dreyfus GD, Corbi PJ, Chan KM, et al. Secondary tricuspid regurgitation or dilatation: which should be the criteria for surgical repair? Ann Thorac Surg 2005;79(1):127–32.

[46] McCarthy PM, Bhudia SK, Rajeswaran J, et al. Tricuspid valve repair: durability and risk factors for failure. J Thorac Cardiovasc Surg 2004;127(3):674–85.

[47] Power JM, Raman J, Dornom A, et al. Passive ventricular constraint amends the course of heart failure: a study in an ovine model of dilated cardiomyopathy. Cardiovasc Res 1999;44(3):549–55.

[48] Chaudhry PA, Mishima T, Sharov VG, et al. Passive epicardial containment prevents ventricular remodeling in heart failure. Ann Thorac Surg 2000;70(4):1275–80.

[49] Konertz WF, Shapland JE, Hotz H, et al. Passive containment and reverse remodeling by a novel textile cardiac support device. Circulation 2001; 104(12 Suppl 1):I270–5.

[50] Maisano F, Redaelli A, Soncini M, et al. An annular prosthesis for the treatment of functional mitral regurgitation: finite element model analysis of a dog bone-shaped ring prosthesis. Ann Thorac Surg 2005;79(4):1268–75.

[51] Cribier A, Eltchaninoff H, Tron C, et al. Percutaneous implantation of aortic valve prosthesis in patients with calcific aortic stenosis: technical advances, clinical results and future strategies. J Interv Cardiol 2006;19(5 Suppl):S87–96.

[52] Grube E, Laborde JC, Gerckens U, et al. Percutaneous implantation of the CoreValve self-expanding valve prosthesis in high-risk patients with aortic valve disease: the Siegburg first-in-man study. Circulation 2006;114(15):1616–24.

[53] Khambadkone S, Coats L, Taylor A, et al. Percutaneous pulmonary valve implantation in humans: results in 59 consecutive patients. Circulation 2005; 112(8):1189–97.

ELSEVIER
SAUNDERS

Heart Failure Clin 3 (2007) 299–315

HEART
FAILURE
CLINICS

Patients who Have Dilated Cardiomyopathy Must Have a Trial of Bridge to Recovery (Pro)

Johannes Mueller, MD[a],*, Gerd Wallukat, PhD[b]

[a]Berlin Heart, Berlin, Germany
[b]Max Delbrueck Center, Berlin, Germany

Healing of idiopathic dilated cardiomyopathy (IDC) by drug therapy has not yet been successful. Mechanical unloading of the heart by an assist device is the only available measure that allows the heart a period of relative rest in which functional improvement may be achieved by interrupting the vicious circle of increasing wall tension and functional impairment. The hearts of a subset of patients who have IDC improve to normal or near-normal function when supported by a device. It is believed that under unloading conditions, special medical supplementation may enhance the process of improvement [1–9].

End-stage heart failure in patients who have dilated cardiomyopathy is characterized by volume and pressure overload of the left and/or right ventricle. The ventricular wall and the interventricular septum are stretched and therefore thinned. The myocardial structure is severely disturbed by a collagen composition of the extracellular matrix that is out of balance [10–12]. Arrhythmia and conductance disturbances are the consequence. Finally, because of the inability of the heart to pump a sufficient volume of blood to the end organs, a globally impaired supply with oxygen is the result. Medically, these patients are treated with full antifailure medication, which, after a time of improvement, cannot avoid a trend toward further deterioration in most patients [13,14]. Likewise the application of devices with biventricular pacing capability postpones the process of deterioration but does not lead to long-term sustained improvement of cardiac function. At this stage, cardiac transplantation is the logical next step to keep the patient alive. However, if a donor heart is not available, the *ultima ratio* is the implantation of a mechanical cardiac assist system, which leads to an immediate improvement of the overall oxygen supply and of end-organ function [15,16].

Because the number of donor organs is limited and indeed has even decreased within the past years, there is growing significance attached to the application of mechanical assist devices as a method to save the lives of patients who are facing imminent death [17].

The development of cardiac assist devices has made much progress within the last 10 years. In the 1980s, mainly paracorporeal devices were available; however, in the 1990s, the partly implantable and fully implantable pulsatile cardiac support systems emerged and played an increasing role (Fig. 1) [18,19]. Then, in 1998, the first rotary blood pump was implanted [20]. Rotary pumps are significantly smaller, free of noise, and have lower power consumption than the pulsatile devices (Fig. 2). Most of these devices are placed above the diaphragm and do not need a pocket between two abdominal muscle layers [21–23]. With these new devices, the assist device technology has reached a status whereby the surgical implantation procedure is easier than with the former systems, and infection —one of the critical problems related to the size of the devices—no longer plays a prominent role. The remaining problem with these pumps alludes to thromboembolic events and potentially long-term effects caused by the reduced pulsatility of the blood

* Corresponding author. Berlin Heart, Wiesenweg 10, 12247 Berlin, Germany.
  E-mail address: johannes.mueller@berlinheart.de (J. Mueller).

1551-7136/07/$ - see front matter © 2007 Elsevier Inc. All rights reserved.
doi:10.1016/j.hfc.2007.05.006

heartfailure.theclinics.com

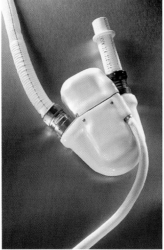 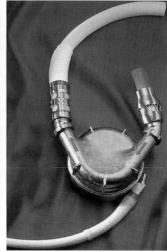

Fig. 1. The pulsatile devices Novacor N 100 LVAS from Worldheart (*left*). This device can be adjusted to a full-to-empty mode, to a synchronized mode and to a fixed rate mode. In the synchronized mode, maximum unloading of the left ventricle will be achieved. The pulsatile HeartMate 1 VE cardiac assist system from Thoratec (*right*). The HeartMate 1 has two operational modes: a fixed rate mode and an automatic mode (full-to-empty mode). Both modes are in asynchrony to the heartbeat. Random synchrony of the pump and the heart may occur.

flow and pressure. The overall risk that the patients have to take is now lower, with the consequence that these devices can be implanted in patients in an earlier stage of the disease.

This article describes the favorable effects on ventricular function over time after placement of a left ventricular assist device (LVAD) and experience with weaning from the LVAD without performing transplantation and outlines the potential benefit for the patients. Preconditions for an optimal improvement of cardiac performance and observations of changes on the molecular level caused by decompression are discussed.

Comparing this with older articles, the reader who has followed the progress in this area of medicine will note some changes in the description and assessment of LVAD application. This is due to the availability of a new generation of devices and the continuous learning process to which LVAD medicine is subject. However, since the author's own first report on successful weaning of a group of four patients who had dilated cardiomyopathy from an LVAD was published in 1996, not much progress has been made with regard to the questions that arose then about the pathophysiologic nature of heart failure, its reversibility, and the significance of chronic or viral myocarditis as a trigger for IDC [1,24–26]. In European clinical reality, most patients receive their LVAD as a bridging device to transplantation,

and only several weeks after placement, a decision about weaning can be made [27]. Due to reasons that are not discussed here, in the United States, the decision for the intention of a device placement has to be made before implantation. Additionally, there is still no parameter available that allows estimation of how long the improved cardiac function will persist.

Preconditions for weaning

Although support of the patient's hemodynamic condition is the primary goal of LVAD placement, a significant unloading of the ventricle in the postoperative phase is a precondition for achieving functional cardiac improvement.

The application of an LVAD leads to decompression of the left ventricle with reduction of the intraventricular volume and pressure. The ventricle wall tension drops dramatically, and perfusion of the myocardium normalizes [28–30]. Although none of the available devices provide information on the amount of pressure reduction, from clinical observations it seems to be plausible that the resulting pressure is at least partially dependent on the LVAD used and the mode of operation. Devices pumping in synchrony with the cardiac cycle are able to eject blood during diastole (diastolic counterpulsation), which results in an optimal unloading of the ventricle and perfusion of the coronary

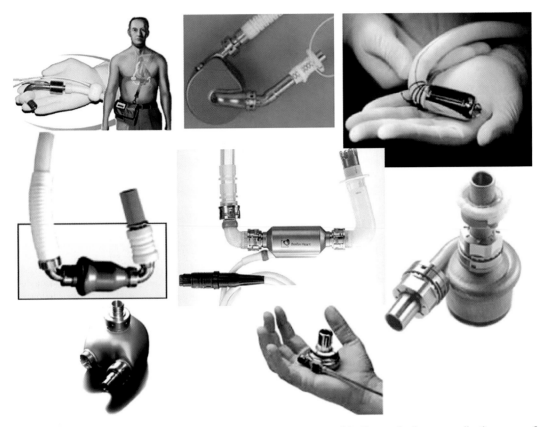

Fig. 2. Several available rotary blood pumps. Most of them are approved in Europe for human application, none of them in the United States. *From the left upper corner to the right lower corner:* the Micromed Debakey VAD from Micromed Cardiovasular, the Duraheart from Terumo Heart, the INCOR from Berlin Heart, the HeartMate II from Thoratec, the Jarvic 2000 FlowMaker from Jarvic Heart, the Coraide LVAD from Arrow, the Ventrassist from Ventracor, and the HVAD from Heartware.

vessels [31]. A full-to-empty or automatic operation mode randomly leads to good drainage too but also to a high intraventricular pressure when pump and heart eject blood at the same moment. This results in isometric ventricular contraction, which is highly consumptive of energy and can cause excessive stretching of the myocardium [32,33]. Therefore, devices or cannula positions (ie, in the atrium) that do not reach a significant pressure and volume unloading most likely do not lead to an improvement of cardiac function. This applies also to systems that are named *true assist devices* because they unload only the ventricle volume to a certain degree, which may not be sufficient to achieve a significant pressure reduction. In principle, rotary blood pumps, if they are powerful enough for a particular patient, have the potential to unload the heart continuously during systole and diastole, leading to overall unloading of the heart, which, however, if they cannot provide sufficient flow

against a given pressure, may not be as pronounced as the unloading with displacement pumps, in particular with the Novacor device [34].

Treatment after device placement

In the early era of LVAD application, treatment of patients with antifailure medication was considered to be unnecessary because the goal was transplantation, not an improvement of the heart function.

After improvement of cardiac function by unloading was accepted to be not only an effect for the short term but a serious option for patients who had heart failure, the behavior of the treating physicians in this respect changed; in fact it became reversed. The question that arose was how patients can be medically treated to intensify the cardiac improvement especially as every patient who has IDC who needs LVAD placement is a potential candidate for weaning and has to be treated accordingly [35–38].

After patients have left the intensive care unit and are hemodynamically and physically stabilized, aggressive medical treatment of heart failure is initiated in accordance with the recommendations of the American Heart Association [39,40]. This aims at maximizing unloading as well as having a direct effect on component parts of the myocardium to reverse pathologic hypertrophy and normalize cellular metabolic function [35].

This medication includes mainly ACE inhibitors, AT-1 blockers, beta-blockers, aldosterone antagonists, and electrolytes. It aims at attaining afterload reduction and a moderate heart rate, reducing myocardial oxygen demand, and reducing the neurohumoral activation that occurs in parallel with heart failure [41–43]. This treatment is based on the concept that activation of the renin-angiotensin-aldosterone system (RAAS) in heart failure is maladaptive and can be an important cause of remodeling [44,45]. If possible, long-term administration of diuretics should be avoided because, especially in patients who have rotary blood pumps, a sufficient volume status is a precondition for satisfactory flow through the pump. A mean arterial pressure between 75 and 80 mmHg is a favorable condition for pump ejection and, as a positive side effect, reduces the rate of hemolysis.

In the early days of weaning, the additional administration of antioxidants, enzymes (bromelaine, trypsine, rutoside), phospholipids, and fatty acids (omega-3 fatty acids) was regarded as unproven adjuvant supplementation; however, the number of articles has dramatically increased that certify favorable effects on cardiac function and oxidative stress reduction [46–62]. As heart failure per se is correlated with a high degree of oxidative stress, the use of a mechanical assist device enhances that further. According to the still preliminary experience, the nutritional supplementation reduces the number of infections and possibly the number of thromboembolic events, makes the blood cells shear stress resistant, improves the rheology by cell membrane stabilization, and reduces the proinflammatory cytokines [63–65].

Cardiac function following left ventricular assist device implantation

Echocardiography is selected for the assessment of cardiac performance, because it is a noninvasive, easy, and frequently applicable method. To avoid any interobserver variability, all examinations should be performed by the same operator. Left ventricular intracavitary dimensions in diastole (LVIDd) are measured by motion mode, whereas left ventricular ejection fraction (EF) is calculated from two reliable orthogonal views that use the biplanar Simpson's rule approach. Studies are conducted once every 2 to 3 weeks after device implantation [66–69].

With a regularly running pump, if LVEF and LVIDd reveal normalization of cardiac function (LVEF 40%–45%) and dimension (LVIDd 55 mm), the pulsatile pumps are set at the lowest possible pumping frequency. Eventually the pumps are stopped to evaluate the heart without mechanical support.

A different approach has to be selected if rotary pumps are used. Because these generate a negative pressure at their inflow side, the aforementioned precondition for further evaluation is frequently fulfilled as a result of active suction of the pump. Therefore, a shrunk small left ventricle must not necessarily be associated with improvement. Stopping or low rotor speed of a rotary pump, however, leads to retrograde flow of different degrees into the ventricle. Therefore, a realistic assessment of cardiac function can only be made by reducing the rotor speed to a value that results in a zero net flow over the time of one cardiac cycle. With a running axial flow device pumping a zero net flow, if echocardiography reveals normalization, these data can be rated as being an effect of unloading.

In addition to LVIDd and EF, wall motion velocity in systole (Sm), velocity time integration, and strain rate measurements can used as parameters for the assessment of cardiac improvement (Figs. 3 and 4).

Because no completely load-independent index to appropriately measure the contractile state exists, the selected parameters have limitations. LVEF and Sm measurements are load-dependent, but they are widely used and are reproducible across centers. To assess whether the observed increase in LVEF and Sm might be caused by afterload reduction instead of by improvement in the contractile state, the meridional end-systolic wall stress is calculated using cuff systolic blood pressure in a generally accepted and invasively validated formula according to Pouseille's law [70–72].

The impact of preload changes on LVEF and Sm is difficult to assess. However, considering the significant reduction in LVIDd as well as an

Before device placement   After device removal

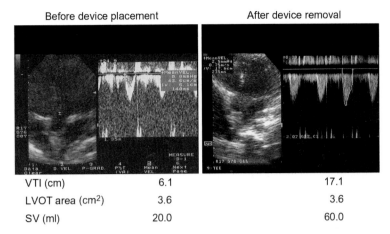

	Before device placement	After device removal
VTI (cm)	6.1	17.1
LVOT area (cm²)	3.6	3.6
SV (ml)	20.0	60.0

Fig. 3. The velocity time integration measured by echocardiography in a patient before device placement and after removal of the system. The velocity time integration has increased from 6.1 to 17.1 cm; from this an increase of the stroke volume (SV) from 20 to 60 mL can be calculated. LVOT: left ventricular outflow tract.

absence of significant changes in transmitral peak E wave velocity and E/A ratio throughout the follow-up period, a significant contribution of preload changes to the increase in LVEF cannot be justifiably assumed either. Although echocardiography enables the measurement of innumerable other parameters that may contribute to a general picture of cardiac performance, LVEF, LVIDd, and some degree Sm, velocity time integration and the strain rate seem sufficient to assess the process of reverse remodeling [73–75].

Process of weaning

If prolonged unloading of the ventricle leads to enhanced development of myocardial atrophy and fibrosis, appropriate adjustment of the pumping mode to the extent allowable by the individual pump settings seems a valuable adjunct in optimizing the recovery process. Although early postoperative maximal unloading of the left ventricle is the goal of every pump, long-term loading of the heart may have benefits thereafter. To reach this goal, the device must be adjusted to the full-to-empty or ideally to a synchronized mode, which leads to a maximal unloading. Loading of the heart can be achieved by reducing the pumping function of the device [33,35].

Running a pulsatile pump in a fixed rate mode randomly leads to synchronization of the heart and the pump and, thereby, to ventricular unloading but, in phases of asynchrony between the heart and the device, the heart can be extremely loaded [35]. The authors' investigations have

Before device placement   After device removal

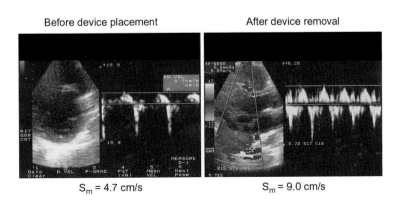

$S_m = 4.7$ cm/s $S_m = 9.0$ cm/s

Fig. 4. The maximum wall motion velocity in systole (Sm) before device implantation and after pump removal measured in the same patient. An increase of nearly 100% is to be seen as the effect of ventricular unloading by the assist device.

shown that an optimally unloaded left ventricle develops pressure values between 40 mmHg and 60 mmHg. However, a loaded ventricle with a pumping rate of 50 bpm produces various pressure values between 40 and 180 mmHg. The provision of an adjustment choice seems appropriate for patients who are potential candidates for device removal.

Because rotary devices behave differently to pulsatile systems, the loading strategy has to be a modified one. Ideally, the flow could be reduced stepwise to zero. However, these devices perform optimally at their so-called design point, which is usually at a flow of approximately 5 L against a pressure of 70 to 80 mmHg. At a flow rate below 2.5 L, the continuous flow inside the pump may be disrupted with the effect of an increasing hemolysis rate, platelet activation, and danger of thrombus formation.

Explantation procedure

An exact description of the procedure has already been published elsewhere [27]. In accordance with the aim to achieve a smooth transition from an unloaded to a loaded heart and to avoid any myocyte destruction, during the explantation procedure, the heart should be kept as undisturbed as possible. The underlying concept is that the myocardium has developed some degree of atrophy during the time of unloading and is extremely sensitive to any additional trauma. Optionally, during the explantation procedure the inflow cannula may remain in place and will be carefully closed by ligation or plugging with a preformed plug. The same can be done with the outflow cannula. In axial flow pumps, which are placed inside the thorax, the outflow cannula can be removed in total.

Great care is taken in restricting volume loading, aiming for a low central venous pressure. The same principle is applied to blood pressure control. A low systemic pressure should be accepted, because it has been learned that blood pressure decreases with pump stoppage but recovers without intervention within a short period of time. To keep blood pressure and heart rate acceptably low, the administration of ACE inhibitors, AT-1 blockers, and/or beta-blockers within hours of surgery might be necessary.

Experience

The experiences described are the result of evolving observations made while dealing with an increasing number of patients. In the early experience, it was believed that maximal unloading of the left heart over as long a period as possible would result in optimal recovery of cardiac function. A detailed analysis of the early data, however, revealed that this approach was not satisfactory. Currently available literature summarizes the different approaches and clinical results obtained in patients who were weaned from devices after having shown functional cardiac improvement [76,77].

An interesting finding was that the relationship between the duration of cardiac unloading and the improvement of LVEF and diameter advanced stepwise over time until a maximum performance was reached. This "optimal" value was not improved with further length of maximal unloading. On the contrary, the longer the unloading of the ventricle lasted, the more the cardiac performance decreased. This was most dramatically seen in patients who remained on the device (fully unloaded) for prolonged periods of time (more than 6 months) and who finally underwent cardiac transplantation. At the time of transplantation, their cardiac performance had approached that seen before LVAD placement, even though they had exhibited an intervening period of improvement. Therefore, it is believed that long-term unloading is a major factor contributing to myocardial atrophy and fibrosis. The authors speculate that a mode of pump operation designed to maximally unload the left ventricle may be the reason for the increased myocardial fibrosis seen at the time of transplantation. The fact that a certain degree of intraventricular pressure is necessary for a balanced gene expression, protein synthesis, and myocardial metabolism has been described [78].

Chronic myocarditis

Controversy surrounds the question of whether cardiac unloading produces genuine myocardial recovery in IDC or whether IDC is a result of chronic myocarditis and cardiac unloading just induces progressive healing of the myocarditis [79–81]. The authors' examinations of tissue specimens revealed that both, patients who have signs of inflammation and who do not have signs of inflammation in the myocardium experienced improvement of function. Therefore, it can be concluded that some patients may recover from chronic myocarditis but that no general rule can be derived that improvement of cardiac function represents only recovery from chronic myocarditis [82].

Changes in biomarkers

The process of deterioration of patients who have heart failure is correlated with a trend toward increasing remodeling of the heart. Different components of the myocardium are involved, including the myocytes, the matrix, the fibroblasts, and the endothelial cells [35,76,77,83–92]. The myocytes change their size with a distinct enlargement of the long axis, which is associated with deterioration in contractile and relaxation function, with the effect of insensitivity to catecholamines and with the induction of a specific gene program involving several groups of genes [35,93–96].

Looking at the literature, one finds descriptions of changes during LVAD support in different biomarkers (eg, in gene expression, different receptor expression, proinflammatory cytokines, complement activation, the composition of extracellular matrix, hormones, enzymes, protein kinases, markers for apoptosis, L-type Ca^{2+} channel density and myocyte histology) [97–110].

The authors' research based on myocardial specimens taken at the time of implantation and removal of the device, it was found a uniform increase in mRNA expression of 17 and a decrease of 26 different genes. This analysis was done with gene microarrays (Affymetrix HG-U133A) that were able to detect the expression of 22,116 genes simultaneously. Out of this huge number, only 43 genes were regulated in the same direction varying between factors of 1.40 and 8.57. This data demonstrate that the gene patterns in the myocardium of different patients are extremely inhomogeneous, although the specimens were taken from the same area of the heart and clinically the patients appeared more or less the same. Additionally, real-time quantitative PCR (TaqMan) of 32 different parameters was performed on the myocardium taken at implantation and explantation, and the results were compared with regard to changes between implantation and removal of the device. For example, expression of beta-1 adrenoceptor, phospholamban, ANP and BNP uniformly showed a significant increase or decrease by unloading, respectively (Figs. 5–8). However, in contrast to what has been described in the literature—mainly based on a small numbers of specimens—and to what one would have expected,

expression of MMP-9, EMMPRIN, SERCA 2A, tryptase, and fibronectin in the myocardium and other parameters increased in some and decreased in other patients. This heterogeneity was confirmed on the protein level. Although the patients from whom the specimens were taken had the same type of assist device and the same mode of operation was applied, the unloading and loading of the left ventricle differed between patients. This may be a possible explanation, but the huge variability may also be due to individual differences between the patients. Although the number of tryptase-positive mast cells did not differ between the myocardium of weaned and nonweaned patients, on the cellular level it could be seen that patients who needed transplantation later on had in their myocardium taken at device placement a significantly higher number of tryptase positive mast cells with degranulation of tryptase compared with the mast cells in the myocardium of patients who could be weaned (Fig. 9).

Changes in the extracellular matrix

There are indicators that the extracellular matrix plays a significant role in heart failure [111–114]. In the normal human myocardium, myocytes constitute 76% of the structural space; 24% of it belongs to the nonmyocyte compartment [115,116]. Two thirds of all cells in the myocardium are nonmyocyte cells. Collagen is the most important component in the extracellular matrix. In volume-overloaded ventricles, the collagen types I and III ratio shifts toward collagen type I and in pressure-overloaded ventricles toward collagen type III [117–125]. The synthesis of collagen undergoes a maturation process from immature collagen fibers to functioning fibers. An analysis of the total collagen and the collagen subfractions (ie, neutral salt collagen [NSC], acid soluble collagen [ASC] and insoluble collagen [ISC]) from three different groups of myocardium was performed to provide information on the rate of collagen synthesis. Myocardium was available from patients at the time of implantation of the device and from the same patients at the time of removal of the device following cardiac transplantation (pre- and post-LVAD transplanted groups). Further, there were myocardial samples taken at the time of device placement from patients who could later be weaned from the device due to sufficient cardiac improvement (weaned group). Before LVAD placement, NSC and ISC in the weaning group were higher

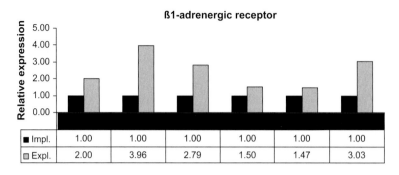

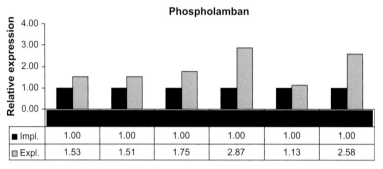

Fig. 5. Gene expression of the beta-1-adrenoceptor and phospholamban in the myocardium of six patients. The specimens were taken at the time of implantation of the device and at transplantation (explantation of the system). The unloading leads to a significant increase of gene expression in all patients.

and ASC in the transplanted group was lower than in controls (myocardium from unused donor hearts). After LVAD implantation total collagen was higher, but ASC was also lower in the transplanted group than in the controls. Comparing the pre- and post-LVAD subgroups of the transplanted and weaning groups, all collagen fraction contents were lower before LVAD implantation in the transplanted group than in the weaning group (Figs. 10 and 11). This difference disappeared during LVAD support. Comparison of the pre- and post-LVAD subgroups of the transplanted groups showed an increase of NSC and total collagen after LVAD support.

To assess the rate of synthesis of collagen type 1 and 3 during the time of mechanical support, the authors analyzed the procollagen PICP and PINP and the procollagen PIIINP from the serum of the patients [126–132]. The changes of serum peptide concentration showed that PIIINP increased constantly in the transplanted patients, but PICP and PINP increased in the weaned patients after LVAD implantation.

Conclusions

There is still intensive discussion of whether weaning is a realistic option for a considerable portion of patients in need of mechanical cardiac support. Excluding from the discussion patients with acute myocarditis or postcardiotomy syndrome who have a high chance for cardiac improvement in accordance with the nature of their diseases, most groups remain skeptical with regard to the long-term success of this measure. Indeed the number of patients who could be successfully weaned is still small. This fact is even more pronounced by the observation during the last couple of years that patients who are supported by rotary pumps show a lower degree of unloading with the consequence of a minor level of functional improvement and a reduced number of weaned patients, probably, because the myocardial inflammation cannot be overcome.

Thus, although the number of patients and the follow-up period are still limited, comparison of the weaning data with the results after cardiac transplantation shows that these are strikingly similar. The success may depend on the intensive treatment of heart failure concomitant to the significant unloading of the heart as described, and on the policy that every patient who has a device is a potential candidate for weaning, which gives rise to frequent close examinations of the cardiac function.

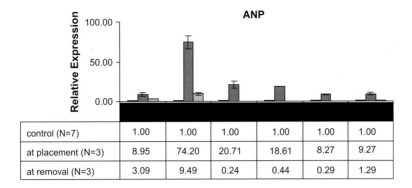

control (N=7)	1.00	1.00	1.00	1.00	1.00	1.00
at placement (N=3)	8.95	74.20	20.71	18.61	8.27	9.27
at removal (N=3)	3.09	9.49	0.24	0.44	0.29	1.29

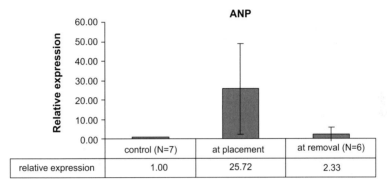

	control (N=7)	at placement	at removal (N=6)
relative expression	1.00	25.72	2.33

Fig. 6. Gene expression of ANP in the myocardium of nonused donor hearts (N = 7, controls) and in the myocardium of patients taken at the time of device placement and transplantation (device removal). The upper panel shows the individual expression in the myocardium of each patient (three measurements per patient) compared with the control tissue and the lower panel the mean values of all patients. There is great interindividual variability in ANP expression—three patients reached ANP values lower than normal; nevertheless, none of the patients could be weaned due to imperfect cardiac function improvement. BNP expression data are similar (data not shown).

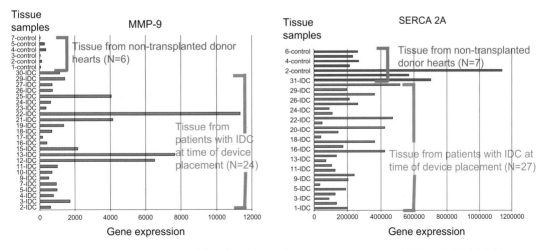

Fig. 7. Two examples of the huge interindividual variability of the gene expression of MMP-9 and SERCA 2A in myocardium from nonused donor hearts and from patients who had IDC at the time of assist device implantation. Cardiac function improvement in the 24/27 patients from whom the specimens were taken was sufficient to justify weaning in all later on.

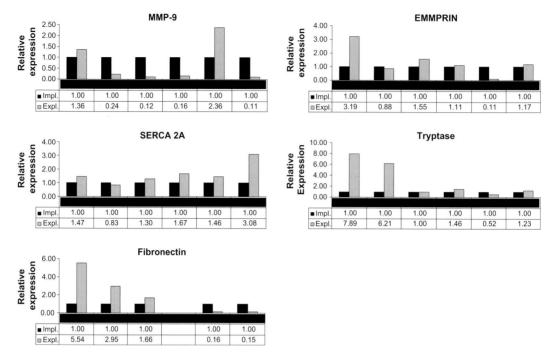

Fig. 8. Five more examples of the lack of uniformity of gene expression in the myocardium of MMP-9, EMMPRIN, SERCA 2A, tryptase, and fibronectin in patients all exposed to left ventricular unloading by a pulsatile assist device. The specimens were all taken at the time of device placement, and none of the patients could be weaned.

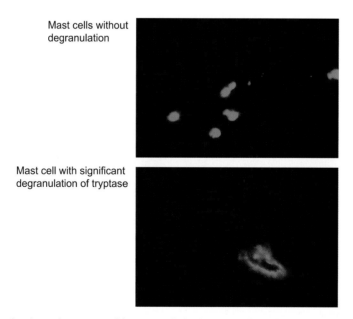

Fig. 9. Immunohistochemistry of tryptase positive mast cells in the myocardium of patients who could be weaned from the device due to improvement of cardiac function (*upper panel*) and who could not be weaned (*lower panel*) because improvement was not sufficient. The tissue was taken at the time of device implantation. Degranulation of tryptase is obvious in the lower panel. There is no degranulation in the upper. Tryptase influences the process of fibrosis in the myocardium.

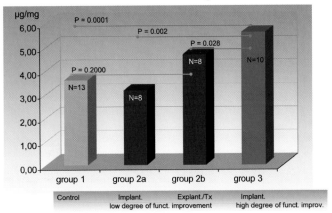

Fig. 10. This histogram shows the mean Neutral Soluble Collagen (NSC) content in several groups. Compared with group 1 (ie, the control group), the NSC of group 2a (ie, in the myocardium of the patients who showed only little functional cardiac improvement by mechanical unloading) is statistically not different. However, after unloading (group 2b), at the time of transplantation and device removal, NSC is increased significantly. In the myocardium of patients who revealed significant functional improvement so that weaning was possible and transplantation was not longer indicated, NSC was already at the time of device implantation significantly higher than in the control group 1, and groups 2a and b.

Furthermore, because the use of implantable displacement pumps is significantly decreased within the last couple of years and rotary blood pumps are the mainly applied pumps, the number of patients who show functional improvement dropped clearly. This is obviously caused by the fact that rotary blood pumps unload the ventricle to a lesser amount with the consequence of a less pronounced improvement.

On the one hand many groups have observed that improvements on the molecular level were frequently not paralleled by pronounced functional improvement. On the other hand functional improvement could not be confirmed on the

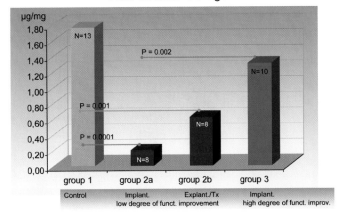

Fig. 11. The distribution of the acid soluble collagen (ASC) between the groups looks similar as in Fig. 10 displayed. ASC is high in the control group, group 1, and significantly lower in the myocardium of patients of group 2a, at the time of device placement. Unloading leads to a pronounced increase of ASC, which is, however, statistically not significant between group 2a and b. Patients who could be weaned later on due to functional cardiac improvement, revealed that at the time of device placement already ASC was high, significantly higher than in group 2a and b and not significantly different to the control group values.

molecular level. This may explain the enormous heterogeneity in the gene expression data between the patients. It may also mean that the observed molecular changes represent the process of adaptation to impaired cardiac function. This process seems to be independent of the original disease, which may be similar among the patients. Furthermore, the placement of a cardiac assist device came too late to initiate a reverse remodeling process due to a maladaption process, which had already masked the disease. These reflections are in accordance with the observation that patients who have a short history of heart failure have a significantly better chance of cardiac recovery.

It cannot be excluded that the type of assist device used, the mode of operation, and the degree of unloading or loading may influence the improvement process and may be responsible for the great variety in the results published. The same assist device running in the same mode may have different effects on the degree of decompression of the heart and on the changes in the myocardial structure.

Changes in myocardial collagen content considered as a sign of myocardial interstitial remodeling are definite in IDC. The changes involve not total collagen but the collagen fraction. The changes in myocardial collagen content in IDC are not identical: NSC and ISC are increased in the weaned patients; ASC is decreased in the patients following transplantation. Therefore it is considered that the increase in NSC and ISC may be related to good prognosis and the decrease of ASC to poorer prognosis. It was confirmed that cardiac function is improved after LVAD support. As cardiac function improved, the collagen and NSC increased simultaneously, so that the changes in collagen could be regarded as an expression of the reverse maladaptive myocardial interstitial remodeling. The changes of serum markers of collagen type I and type III could be continuously observed during LVAD support. The level of PINP and PICP increased in early stages of LVAD support in the weaning group. Therefore, the increases of PINP and PICP representing collagen type I synthesis may be signs of reversion of maladaptive remodeling. However, the constant increase of PIIINP representing collagen type III synthesis may relate to poorer prognosis.

Preview

Since the first patient in 1995 could be weaned, a new generation of cardiac assist devices—the rotary blood pumps—has been introduced in the treatment of heart failure. According to the still limited clinical experience with these pumps, patients who have these devices overcome the inflammatory status related to chronic heart failure not as fast and not as extensively as those who have the pulsatile systems. Furthermore, infectious complications in patients who have rotary pumps are rare because of the small size of the system and the thin and flexible transcutaneous line. This may be a good precondition for recovery provided sufficient unloading of the heart can be obtained, which, however, is probably not the case.

None of the available devices are designed to support recovery. There are no features integrated into the systems that provide the user with information on the degree of unloading. If recovery is to become a real option for a greater number of patients and if this option is to be more independent of random observation, the technologic development of the devices should take this into account by providing the user with exact data on the degree of unloading, the pressure inside the ventricle, and the volume status of the patient. To optimize unloading of the heart in patients who have rotary blood pumps they should capable of sensing the pressure inside the ventricle and adjust the flow accordingly. Further methods with the intention to improve cardiac function while the heart is unloaded are emerging at the horizon. Thus, in animal trials, it could be demonstrated that the application of electrical microcurrent to a diseased heart normalized the extracellular matrix and balanced the collagen components in the myocardium.

Summary

This article documents the experience that mechanical unloading of a diseased heart by LVAD application with the consequence of functional improvement and weaning thereafter is a realistic option. The patient who has been weaned first is still doing fine with sufficient and stable cardiac function since now more than 10 years after device removal. Furthermore, it was discussed how to identify potential patients for weaning, what problems may arise, how the follow-up should be designed, the medication before and after weaning, the surgical procedure and the general management.

It has been discussed why weaning may have failed and the potential reasons for recurrence of heart failure. Since the possibility of weaning can be identified within the first 2 to 3 months after implantation, weaned patients do not have to take the risk of an extended period on a device before transplantation. This is always linked to the possibility of thromboembolism or bleeding even if these are unlikely events with the new generation of devices.

The search for biomarkers that allow predictive assessment of recovery before device implantation has not so far been successful. Procollagen measured in the serum of patients was shown for the first time to be potentially such a parameter.

Comparing the results of the published weaning experience with those of patients following heart transplantation after placement of a cardiac assist device reveals that the results are similar. This comparison excludes, however, aspects such as quality of life, cost-effectiveness, and, most importantly, the saving of a donor heart for another patient.

It could be demonstrated that in the case of recurrence of heart failure, transplantation is still an option, so that the time saved for patients after device removal and before heart failure recurs represents a gain in life time.

Acknowledgment

We are deeply grateful to Dr. Michael Jurmann who provided us with the Figs. 3, 4, 10, and 11. Furthermore, we are very appreciative to Dr. Peter Ellinghaus who performed in a joint research project the micro array analysis and the RT quantitative PCR (Taqman), and designed the accordant figures. Additionally, we are indebted to all patients who gave permission to the analysis of their tissue to support efforts to achieve novel insights into the origin of heart failure.

References

[1] Müller J, Wallukat G, Weng YG, et al. Weaning from mechanical cardiac support in patients with idiopathic dilated cardiomyopathy. Circulation 1997;96(2):542–9.

[2] Rose EA, Frazier OH. Resurrection after mechanical circulatory support. Circulation 1997;96(2): 393–5.

[3] Oz MC, Argenziano M, Catanese KA, et al. Are they an alternative to transplantation? Circulation 1997;95(7):1844–52.

[4] Mancini DM, Beniaminovitz A, Levin H, et al. Low incidence of myocardial recovery after left ventricular assist device implantation in patients with chronic heart failure. Circulation 1998; 98(22):2383–9.

[5] McCarthy PM, Smedira NO, Vargo RL, et al. One hundred patients with the HeartMate left ventricular assist device: evolving concepts and technology. J Thorac Cardiovasc Surg 1998; 115(4):904–12.

[6] Loebe M, Muller J, Hetzer R. Ventricular assistance for recovery of cardiac failure. Curr Opin Cardiol 1999;14(3):234–48.

[7] Hetzer R, Muller J, Weng Y, et al. Cardiac recovery in dilated cardiomyopathy by unloading with a left ventricular assist device. Ann Thorac Surg 1999; 68(2):742–9.

[8] Levin HR, Oz MC, Catanese KA, et al. Transient normalization of systolic and diastolic function after support with a left ventricular assist device in a patient with dilated cardiomyopathy. J Heart Lung Transplant 1996;15(8):840–2.

[9] Levin HR, Oz MC, Chen JM, et al. Reversal of chronic ventricular dilation in patients with end_stage cardiomyopathy by prolonged mechanical unloading. Circulation 1995;91(11):2717–20.

[10] Prockop DJ, Kivirikko KI, Tuderman L, et al. The biosynthesis of collagen and its disorders (first of two parts). N Engl J Med 1979;301(1):13–23.

[11] Prockop DJ, Kivirikko KI, Tuderman L, et al. The biosynthesis of collagen and its disorders (second of two parts). N Engl J Med 1979;301(2):77–85.

[12] Marijianowski MM, Teeling P, Mann J, et al. Dilated cardiomyopathy is associated with an increase in the type I/type III collagen ratio: a quantitative assessment. J Am Coll Cardiol 1995;25(6): 1263–72.

[13] Hall SA, Cigarroa CG, Marcoux L, et al. Time course of improvement in left ventricular function, mass and geometry in patients with congestive heart failure treated with beta-adrenergic blockade. J Am Coll Cardiol 1995; 25(5):1154–61.

[14] Greenberg B, Quinones MA, Koilpillai C, et al. Effects of long-term enalapril therapy on cardiac structure and function in patients with left ventricular dysfunction. Results of the SOLVD echocardiography substudy. Circulation 1995; 91(10):2573–81.

[15] Dasse KA, Frazier OH, Lesniak JM, et al. Clinical responses to ventricular assistance versus transplantation in a series of bridge to transplant patients. ASAIO J 1992;38(3):M622–6.

[16] DeRose JJ Jr, Umana JP, Argenziano M, et al. Implantable left ventricular assist devices provide an excellent outpatient bridge to transplantation and recovery. J Am Coll Cardiol 1997;30(7): 1773–7.

[17] Hertz MI, Taylor DO, Trulock EP, et al. The registry of the international society for heart and lung transplantation: nineteenth official report-2002. J Heart Lung Transplant 2002;21(9):950–70.

[18] Hung TC, Butter DB, Yie CL, et al. Effects of long_term Novacor artificial heart support on blood rheology. ASAIO Trans 1991;37(3):M312–3.

[19] McGee MG, Myers TJ, Abou-Awdi N, et al. Extended support with a left ventricular assist device as a bridge to heart transplantation. ASAIO Trans 1991;37(3):M425–6.

[20] Noon GP, Morley D, Irwin S, et al. Development and clinical application of the MicroMed DeBakey VAD. Curr Opin Cardiol 2000;15(3):166–71.

[21] Siegenthaler MP, Martin J, van de Loo A, et al. Implantation of the permanent Jarvik-2000 left ventricular assist device: a single-center experience. J Am Coll Cardiol 2002;39(11):1764–72.

[22] Christiansen S, Van Aken H, Breithardt GG, et al. Successful cardiac transplantation after 4 cases of DeBakey left ventricular assist device failure. J Heart Lung Transplant 2002;21(6):706–9.

[23] Westaby S, Frazier OH, Beyersdorf F, et al. The Jarvik 2000 Heart. Clinical validation of the intraventricular position. Eur J Cardiothorac Surg 2002; 22(2):228–32.

[24] Pankuweit S, Hufnagel G, Eckhardt H, et al. Cardiotropic DNA viruses and bacteria in the pathogenesis of dilated cardiomyopathy with or without inflammation. Med Klin 1998;93(4):223–8.

[25] Mahon NG, Zal B, Arno G, et al. Absence of viral nucleic acids in early and late dilated cardiomyopathy. Heart 2001;86(6):687–92.

[26] Klein RM, Vester EG, Brehm MU, et al. Inflammation of the myocardium as an arrhythmia trigger. Z Kardiol 2000;89(Suppl 3):24–35.

[27] Mueller J, Hetzer R. Left ventricular recovery during left ventricular assist device support. In: Goldstein DJ, Oz MC, editors. Cardiac assist devices. Armonk (NY): Futura Publishing Company; 2000. p. 121–36.

[28] Hendry PJ, Masters RG, Mussivand TV, et al. Circulatory support for cardiogenic shock due to acute myocardial infarction: a Canadian experience. Can J Cardiol 1999;15(10):1090–4.

[29] Sukehiro S, Flameng W. Effects of left ventricular assist for cardiogenic shock on cardiac function and organ blood flow distribution. Ann Thorac Surg 1990;50(3):374–83.

[30] Miyama M. Renal, intestinal and whole body metabolic changes in pig LVAD model. Hokkaido Igaku Zasshi 1999;74(4):331–7.

[31] Tevaearai HT, Mueller XM, Jegger D, et al. Atrial, ventricular, or both cannulation sites to optimize left ventricular assistance? ASAIO J 2001;47(3): 261–5.

[32] Yacoub MH, Tansley P, Birks EJ, et al. A novel combination therapy to revers end-stage heart failure. Transplantation Proceedings 2001;33: 2762–4.

[33] Maybaum S, Williams M, Barbone A, et al. Assessment of synchrony relationships between the native left ventricle and the HeartMate left ventricular assist device. J Heart Lung Transplant 2002;21(5): 509–15.

[34] Hetzer R, Weng Y, Potapov EV, et al. First experiences with a novel magnetically suspended axial flow left ventricular assist device. Eur J Cardiothorac Surg 2004;25(6):964–70.

[35] Yacoub MH. A novel strategy to maximize the efficacy of left ventricular assist devices as bridge to recovery. Eur Heart J 2002;22:534–40.

[36] Wong K, Boheler KR, Petrou M, et al. Pharmacological modulation of pressure-overload cardiac hypertrophy: changes in ventricular function, extracellular matrix, and gene expression. Circulation 1997;96(7):2239–46.

[37] Wong K, Boheler KR, Bishop J, et al. Clenbuterol induces cardiac hypertrophy with normal functional, morphological and molecular features. Cardiovasc Res 1998;37(1):115–22.

[38] Weber KT. Targeting pathological remodelling: concepts of cardioprotection and reparation. Circulation 200(102):1342–45.

[39] Hunt SA, Baker DW, Chin MH, et al. American College of Cardiology/American Heart Association Task Force on Practice Guidelines (Committee to Revise the 1995 Guidelines for the Evaluation and Management of Heart Failure).; International Society for Heart and Lung Transplantation.; Heart Failure Society of America. ACC/ AHA guidelines for the evaluation and management of chronic heart failure in the adult: executive summary. A report of the American College of Cardiology/American Heart Association Task Force on Practice Guidelines (Committee to revise the 1995 guidelines for the evaluation and management of heart failure): developed in collaboration with the International Society for Heart and Lung Transplantation; endorsed by the Heart Failure Society of America. Circulation 2001;104(24):2996–3007.

[40] Ahmed A. American College of Cardiology/American Heart Association. Chronic heart failure evaluation and management guidelines: relevance to the geriatric practice. J Am Geriatr Soc 2003; 51(1):123–6.

[41] Beuckelmann DJ. [Hormonal hyperactivity in heart failure. Differences in beta blockers]. Herz 2002;27(Suppl 1):9–15 [in German].

[42] Stanek B, Frey B, Hulsmann M, et al. Prognostic evaluation of neurohumoral plasma levels before and during beta-blocker therapy in advanced left ventricular dysfunction. J Am Coll Cardiol 2001;38(2):436–42.

[43] Aronson D, Burger AJ. Effect of beta-blockade on autonomic modulation of heart rate and neurohormonal profile in decompensated heart failure. Ann Noninvasive Electrocardiol 2001;6(2):98–106.

[44] Willenbrock R, Philipp S, Mitrovic V, et al. Neurohumoral blockade in CHF management. J Renin Angiotensin Aldosterone Syst 2000;1(Suppl 1): 24–30.

[45] Brilla CG, Rupp H, Funck R, et al. The renin-angiotensin-aldosterone system and myocardial collagen matrix remodelling in congestive heart failure. Eur Heart J 1995;16(Suppl O):107–9.

[46] Barnes PJ. Therapy of chronic obstructive pulmonary disease. Pharmacol Ther 2003;97(1):87–94.

[47] Landmesser U, Spiekermann S, Dikalov S, et al. Vascular oxidative stress and endothelial dysfunction in patients with chronic heart failure: role of xanthine-oxidase and extracellular superoxide dismutase. Circulation 2002;106(24):3073–8.

[48] Kumar D, Lou H, Singal PK. Oxidative stress and apoptosis in heart dysfunction. Herz 2002;27(7):662–8.

[49] Sun Y, Zhang J, Lu L, et al. Aldosterone-induced inflammation in the rat heart: role of oxidative stress. Am J Pathol 2002;161(5):1773–81.

[50] Nakamura R, Egashira K, Machida Y, et al. Probucol attenuates left ventricular dysfunction and remodeling in tachycardia-induced heart failure: roles of oxidative stress and inflammation. Circulation 2002;106(3):362–7.

[51] Farquharson CA, Butler R, Hill A, et al. Allopurinol improves endothelial dysfunction in chronic heart failure. Circulation 2002;106(2):221–6.

[52] Doehner W, Schoene N, Rauchhaus M, et al. Effects of xanthine oxidase inhibition with allopurinol on endothelial function and peripheral blood flow in hyperuricemic patients with chronic heart failure: results from 2 placebo_controlled studies. Circulation 2002;105(22):2619–24.

[53] Nakamura K, Kusano K, Nakamura Y, et al. Carvedilol decreases elevated oxidative stress in human failing myocardium. Circulation 2002;105(24):2867–71.

[54] Zafari AM, Harrison DG. Free radicals in heart failure: therapeutic targets for old and new drugs. Congest Heart Fail 2002;8(3):129–30.

[55] Sawyer DB, Siwik DA, Xiao L, et al. Role of oxidative stress in myocardial hypertrophy and failure. J Mol Cell Cardiol 2002;34(4):379–88.

[56] Yap CL, Anderson KE, Hughan SC, et al. Essential role for phosphoinositide 3-kinase in shear-dependent signaling between platelet glycoprotein Ib/V/IX and integrin alpha(IIb)beta(3). Blood 2002;99(1):151–8.

[57] Vogel J, Bendas G, Bakowsky U, et al. The role of glycolipids in mediating cell adhesion: a flow chamber study. Biochim Biophys Acta 1998;1372(2):205–15.

[58] Ho M, Maple C, Bancroft A, et al. The beneficial effects of omega_3 and omega_6 essential fatty acid supplementation on red blood cell rheology. Prostaglandins Leukot Essent Fatty Acids 1999;61(1):13–7.

[59] Westerveld HT, de Graaf JC, van Breugel HH, et al. Effects of low-dose EPA-E on glycemic control, lipid profile, lipoprotein(a), platelet aggregation, viscosity, and platelet and vessel wall interaction in NIDDM. Diabetes Care 1993;16(5):683–8.

[60] Ernst E. Effects of n-3 fatty acids on blood rheology. J Intern Med Suppl 1989;225(731):129–32.

[61] Cartwright IJ, Pockley AG, Galloway JH, et al. The effects of dietary omega-3 polyunsaturated fatty acids on erythrocyte membrane phospholipids, erythrocyte deformability and blood viscosity in healthy volunteers. Atherosclerosis 1985;55(3):267–81.

[62] Di Carlo A, Passi S, Ippolito F, et al. Free radical scavenger activity of rutosides. Minerva Cardioangiol 2002;50(6):701–7.

[63] Tretjakovs P, Kalnins U, Dabina I, et al. Nitric oxide production and arachidonic acid metabolism in platelet membranes of coronary heart disease patients with and without diabetes. Med Princ Pract 2003;12(1):10–6.

[64] Kudo I, Murakami M. Phospholipase A2 enzymes. Prostaglandins Other Lipid Mediat 2002;68–9, 3–58.

[65] Weyrich AS, Prescott SM, Zimmerman GA. Platelets, endothelial cells, inflammatory chemokines, and restenosis: complex signaling in the vascular play book. Circulation 2002;106(12):1433–5.

[66] Feigenbaum H. Echocardiographic evaluation of cardiac chambers. In: Feigenbaum H, editor. Echocardiography. Philadelphia: Lea & Febiger; 1994. p. 134–80.

[67] Lejemtel TH, Sonnenblick EH, Frishmann W. Diagnosis and management of heart failure. In: Alexander RW, Schlant RC, Fuster V, editors. Hursts the heart. 9th edition. New York: McGraw-Hill; 1998. p. 745–81.

[68] Feigenbaum H. Echocardiographic examination of the left ventricle. Circulation 1975;51:1–7.

[69] Feigenbaum H. Echocardiography. In: Braunwald E, editor. Heart disease. 4th edition. Philadelphia: W.B. Saunders Co.; 1992. p. 64–115.

[70] Vuille C, Weyman AE. Left ventricle I. General considerations, assessment of chamber size and function. In: Weyman AE, editor. Principles an practice of echocardiography. 2nd edition. Philadelphia: Lea & Febiger; 1994. p. 557–624.

[71] De Simone G, Devereux RB, Roman MJ, et al. Assessment of left ventricular function by the midwall fractional shortening/end-systolic stress relation in human hypertension. J Am Coll Cardiol 1994;23:1444–51.

[72] Reichek N, Wilson J, St. John Sutton M, et al. Noninvasive determination of left ventricular end systolic stress: validation of the method and initial application. Circulation 1982;65:99–108.

[73] Aurigemma GP, Douglass PS, Gaasch WH. Quantitative evaluation of left ventricular structure, wall stress and systolic function. In: Otto CM, editor. The practice of clinical echocardiography. Philadelphia: W.B. Saunders Co.; 1997. p. 1–24.

[74] Hurrell DG, Nishimura RA, Istrup DM, et al. Utility of preload alteration in assessment of ventricular filling pressure by Doppler echocardiography: a simultaneous characterization and Doppler echocardiographic study. J Am Coll Cardiol 1997;30: 459–67.

[75] Lewis JF. Doppler and two-dimensional echocardiographic evaluation in acute and long-term management of the heart failure patient. In: Otto CM, editor. The practice of clinical echocardiography. Philadelphia: W.B. Saunders Co.; 1997. p. 433–48.

[76] Birks EJ, Tansley PD, Hardy J, et al. Left ventricular assist device and drug therapy for the reversal of heart failure. N Engl J Med 2006;355:1873–84.

[77] Dandel M, Weng Y, Siniawski H, et al. Long-term results in patients after weaning from left ventricular assist device. Circulation 2005;112(Suppl I): I-37–45.

[78] Nadruz W Jr, Kobarg CB, Constancio SS, et al. Load-induced transcriptional activation of c-jun in rat myocardium: regulation by myocyte enhancer factor 2. Circ Res 2003;92(2):243–51.

[79] Takeda N. Cardiomyopathy: molecular and immunological aspects [review]Int J Mol Med 2003;11(1): 13–6.

[80] Gauntt C, Huber S. Coxsackievirus experimental heart diseases. Front Biosci 2003;8:E23–35.

[81] Caforio AL, Mahon NJ, Tona F, et al. Circulating cardiac autoantibodies in dilated cardiomyopathy and myocarditis: pathogenetic and clinical significance. Eur J Heart Fail 2002;4(4):411–7.

[82] Kühl U, Schultheiss H-P. What is dilated cardiomyopathy? In: Hetzer R, Hennig E, Loebe M, editors. Mechanical circulatory support. Darmstadt (Germany): Steinkopff Verlag; 1997. p. 69–82.

[83] Katz AM. Cardiomyopathy of overload, a major development of prognosis in congestive heartfailure. N Engl J Med 1990;222:100–10.

[84] Lorrell BH, Carabello BA. Left ventricular hypertrophy pathogenesis, detection and prognosis. Circulation 2000;102:470–9.

[85] Swynghedauw B. Molecular mechanisms of myocardial remodelling. Physiol Rev 1999;79:216–61.

[86] Francis GS. Changing the remodelling process in heart failure. Basic mechanisms and laboratory results. Curr Opin Cardiol 1998;13:156–61.

[87] Hunter JJ, Chien KR. Signalling pathways for cardiac hypertrophy and failure. N Engl J Med 1999; 341:1276–83.

[88] Sugden PH. Signaling in myocardial hypertrophy. Circ Res 1999;84:633–46.

[89] Onodera T, Tamura T, Said S, et al. Maladaptive remodelling of cardiac myocyte shape begins long before failure in hypertension. Hypertension 1998; 32:753–7.

[90] Gerdes AM, Tamura T, Wang X, et al. Myocyte remodelling during the progression to failure in rats with hypertension. Hypertension 1996;28: 604–14.

[91] Gerdes AM, Kellermann SE, Moore JA, et al. Structural remodeling of cardiac myocytes in patients with ischemic cardiomyopathy. Circulation 1992;86(2):426–30.

[92] Gerdes AM, Capasso JM. Structural remodelling and mechanical dysfunction of cardiac myocytes in heart failure. J Mol Cell Cardiol 1995;27: 849–56.

[93] Chien KR. Stress pathways and heart failure. Cell 1999;98:555–8.

[94] Schneider MD, Schwartz RJ. Chips ahoy: gene expression in hearts surveyed by high-density microarrays. Circulation 2000;102:3020–7.

[95] Corbett JM, Why HJ, Wheeler CH, et al. Cardiac protein abnormalities in cardiomyopathy detected by twodimensional polyacrylamide gel electrophoresis. Electrophoresis 1998;19:2031–42.

[96] Latif N, Khan M, Birks E, et al. Upregulation of the Bcl-2 family of proteins in end-stage heart failure. J Am Coll Cardiol 2000;35:1769–77.

[97] Chen X, Piacentino V 3rd, Furukawa S, et al. L-type Ca2+ channel density and regulation are altered in failing human ventricular myocytes and recover after support with mechanical assist devices. Circ Res 2002;91(6):517–24.

[98] de Jonge N, van Wichen DF, Schipper ME, et al. Left ventricular assist device in end-stage heart failure: persistence of structural myocyte damage after unloading. An immunohistochemical analysis of the contractile myofilaments. J Am Coll Cardiol 2002;39(6):963–9.

[99] Milting H, EL-Banayosy A, Kassner A, et al. The time course of natriuretic hormones as plasma markers of myocardial recovery in heart transplant candidates during ventricular assist device support reveals differences among device types. J Heart Lung Transplant 2001;20(9):949–55.

[100] Li YY, Feng Y, McTiernan CF, et al. Downregulation of matrix metalloproteinases and reduction in collagen damage in the failing human heart after support with left ventricular assist devices. Circulation 2001;104(10):1147–52.

[101] Ogletree-Hughes ML, Stull LB, Sweet WE, et al. Mechanical unloading restores beta-adrenergic responsiveness and reverses receptor downregulation in the failing human heart. Circulation 2001;104(8):881–6.

[102] Bruckner BA, Stetson SJ, Perez-Verdia A, et al. Regression of fibrosis and hypertrophy in failing myocardium following mechanical circulatory support. J Heart Lung Transplant 2001;20(4): 457–64.

[103] Arbustini E, Grasso M, Porcu E, et al. Healing of acute myocarditis with left ventricular assist device: morphological recovery and evolution to the aspecific features of dilated cardiomyopathy. Ital Heart J 2001;2(1):55–9.

[104] Bruckner BA, Stetson SJ, Farmer JA, et al. The implications for cardiac recovery of left

ventricular assist device support on myocardial collagen content. Am J Surg 2000;180(6):498–501 [discussion: 501–2].

[105] Mital S, Loke KE, Addonizio LJ, et al. Left ventricular assist device implantation augments nitric oxide dependent control of mitochondrial respiration in failing human hearts. J Am Coll Cardiol 2000;36(6):1897–902.

[106] Torre-Amione G, Stetson SJ, Youker KA, et al. Decreased expression of tumor necrosis factor-alpha in failing human myocardium after mechanical circulatory support: a potential mechanism for cardiac recovery. Circulation 1999;100(11):1189–93.

[107] Loebe M, Gorman K, Burger R, et al. Complement activation in patients undergoing mechanical circulatory support. ASAIO J 1998;44(5):M340–6.

[108] Dipla K, Mattiello JA, Jeevanandam V, et al. Myocyte recovery after mechanical circulatory support in humans with end-stage heart failure. Circulation 1998;97(23):2316–22.

[109] McCarthy PM, Nakatani S, Vargo R, et al. Structural and left ventricular histologic changes after implantable LVAD insertion. Ann Thorac Surg 1995;59(3):609–13.

[110] Birks EJ, Latif N, Bowles C. Measurement of cytokine levels and activation of the apoptotic pathway in patients requiring left ventricular assist device (LVAD): implication for timing of implantation. Circulation 1999;99:2565–70.

[111] Dec GW, Fuster V. Idiopathic dilated cardiomyopathy. N Engl J Med 1994;331:1564–75.

[112] Kopecky SL, Gersh BJ. Dilated cardiomyopathy and myocarditis: natural history, etiology, clinical manifestations, and management. Curr Probl Cardiol 1987;12:573–647.

[113] Pauschinger M, Chandrasekharan K, Li J, et al. Mechanisms of extracellular matrix remodeling in dilated cardiomyopathy. Herz 2002;27:677–82.

[114] Maisch B. Ventricular remodeling. Cardiology 1996;87(Suppl 1):2–10.

[115] Maisch B. Extracellular matrix and cardiac interstitium: restriction is not a restricted phenomenon. Herz 1995;20:75–80.

[116] Frank JS, Langer GA. The myocardial interstitium: its structure and its role in ionic exchange. J Cell Biol 1974;60:586–601.

[117] Weber KT, Janicki JS, Shroff SG, et al. Collagen remodeling of the pressure-overload, hypertrophied non-human primate myocardium. Circ Res 1988;62:757–65.

[118] Li J, Schwimmbeck PL, Tschope C, et al. Collagen degradation in a murine myocarditis model: relevance of matrix metalloproteinase in association with inflammatory induction. Cardiovasc Res 2002;56:235–47.

[119] Spinale FG, Coker ML, Heung LJ, et al. A matrix metalloproteinase induction/activation system exists in the human left ventricular myocardium and is upregulated in heart failure. Circulation 2000;102:1944–9.

[120] Gunja-Smith Z, Morales AR, Romanelli R, et al. Remodeling of human myocardial collagen in idiopathic dilated cardiomyopathy: role of metalloproteinases and pyridinoline cross links. Am J Pathol 1996;148:1639–48.

[121] Spinale FG, Coker ML, Thomas CV, et al. Time-dependent changes in matrix metalloproteinase activity and expression during the progression of congestive heart failure: relation to ventricular and myocyte function. Circ Res 1998;82:482–95.

[122] Spinale FG, Coker ML, Krombach RS, et al. Matrix metalloproteinase inhibition during developing congestive heart failure: effects on left ventricular geometry and function. Circ Res 1999;85:364–76.

[123] Ries C, Petrides PE. Cytokine regulation of matrix metalloproteinase activity and regulatory dysfunction in disease. Biol Chem 1995;376:345–55.

[124] Chancey AL, Brower GL, Peterson JT, et al. Effects of matrix metalloproteinase inhibition on ventricular remodeling due to volume overload. Circulation 2002;105:1983–8.

[125] Thomas CV, Coker ML, Zellner JL, et al. Increased matrix metalloproteinase activity and selective upregulation in LV myocardium from patients with end-stage dilated cardiomyopathy. Circulation 1998;97:1708–15.

[126] Diez J, Laviades C, Mayor G, et al. Increased serum concentration of procollagen peptides in essential hypertension. Relation to cardiac alteration. Circulation 1995;91:1450–6.

[127] Querejeta R, Varo N, Lopez B, et al. Serum carboxy-terminal propeptide of procollagen type I is a marker of myocardial fibrosis in hypertensive heart disease. Circulation 2000;101:1729–35.

[128] Poulsen SH, Høst NB, Jensen SE, et al. Relationship between serum amino-terminal propeptide of type III procollagen and changes of left ventricular function after acute myocardial infarction. Circulation 2000;101:1527–32.

[129] Jensen LT, H-Petersen K, Toft P, et al. Serum aminoterminal type III procollagen peptide reflects repair after acute myocardial infarction. Circulation 1990;81:52–7.

[130] Høst NB, Jensen LT, Bendixen PM, et al. The aminoterminal propeptide of type III procollagen provides new information on prognosis after acute myocardial infarction. Am J Cardiol 1995; 76:869–73.

[131] Sato Y, Kataoka K, Matsumori A, et al. Measuring serum aminoterminal type III procollagen peptide, 7S domain of type IV collagen, and cardiac troponin T in patients with idiopathic dilated cardiomyopathy and secondary cardiomyopathy. Heart 1997;78:505–8.

[132] Klappacher G, Franzen P, Haab D, et al. Measuring extracellular matrix turnover in the serum of patients with idiopathic or ischemic dilated cardiomyopathy and impact on diagnosis and prognosis. Am J Cardiol 1995;75:913–8.

ELSEVIER
SAUNDERS

Heart Failure Clin 3 (2007) 317–319

HEART
FAILURE
CLINICS

Patients Who Have Dilated Cardiomyopathy Must Have a Trial of Bridge to Recovery: The Case Against That Proposition

Philip A. Poole-Wilson, MD, FRCP, FMedSci*

National Heart & Lung Institute, Imperial College London, London, UK

Propositions containing the word "must" are usually mistaken and this proposition is no exception.

In the last few years the management of patients who have severe heart failure has increased in complexity, requiring greater skills and finer judgment from the physician and surgeon. New drugs have emerged, the expertise of physicians in using these drugs has improved, the indications for cardiac transplantation have changed, new surgical techniques have developed, and effective left ventricular assist devices (LVADs) have become available. The newer LVADs are an engineering triumph but raise critical issues regarding how and when they should be used. This problem has been exacerbated by the decline in the number of patients undergoing transplantation, by the dearth of donor hearts, and possibly by a growing public aversion to cardiac transplantation.

Indications for the use of left ventricular assist devices

The availability on the market of many devices to assist the pumping function of the heart has resulted in a new vocabulary. This has led to a surplus of confusion, even misunderstanding, extending from the characteristics and phenotypes of patients and the indications for the use of LVADs to the appropriate assessment of benefit, if any.

The phrase "bridge to recovery" is used to encapsulate the idea that doctors can identify patients who have reversible cardiac dysfunction and who only require transient support of the circulation before spontaneous functional recovery of the heart in situ. Established clinical entities in which this can occur include acute myocarditis, Takotsubo syndrome, acute alcohol ingestion, and depression of cardiac function by toxins or drugs. The phrase might also include patients who have cardiogenic shock attributable to a second group of patients who have myocardial infarction in whom the likely outcome may be transformed. In recent years several authors have possibly identified a third group in which a sizable proportion of patients presenting with severe heart failure of idiopathic origin and with large hearts (dilated cardiomyopathy) do recover spontaneously. These authors have argued that such patients should receive a device pending a decision as to whether to proceed to transplantation. The extent to which this claim is correct is unknown largely because many of these patients may in reality belong to the other two groups of patients.

The phrases "destination treatment" or "life-time therapy" are used to describe the intention at the moment of insertion of the device: that it should remain in place for the life of the patient and that there is no intention to proceed to transplantation. The first such device inserted with this intention was reported in 2000 [1]. Since then many patients around the world have received devices of different designs, although the efficacy remains somewhat uncertain [2,3].

* National Heart & Lung Institute, Imperial College London, Dovehouse Street, London SW3 6LY, United Kingdom.
   E-mail address: p.poole-wilson@imperial.ac.uk

The third phrase in common use is "bridge to transplantation." Here the idea is that by supporting the circulation for a period of time the state of the patient may improve and thus the outcome from transplantation may be enhanced. Serious confusion arises if this group of patients includes both those who have long-term chronic heart failure and those who have acute cardiogenic shock.

Clinical intent

The difficulty with these three phrases is that they do not encapsulate a clear statement of the clinical intention at the time that a decision is made to either undergo transplantation or insert a device. Indeed, these phrases are increasingly misleading at best, and there is an argument for discontinuing their use. For example, a patient having an LVAD inserted as bridge to recovery may not recover and may go on to lifetime therapy or may be deemed suitable for a transplant (ie, bridge to transplantation).

Patients who are likely to die imminently, say within 72 hours, because they have sustained some major cardiac event, present a very different medical problem than patients who have had chronic heart failure for many years with a recent more rapid decline of cardiac function. Furthermore, bridge to recovery is not something that can easily be diagnosed because it is a statement based on a medical judgment about the future prognosis and the diagnosis in a patient. Most physicians specializing in the management of severe heart failure are only too aware of a small group of patients who are often so sick that neither a transplant not a device is considered appropriate, but the patient for one reason or another recovers. The prediction of outcome in severe heart failure is a matter of greater uncertainty than is commonly admitted. To insert an LVAD into a patient, or worse, to transplant a patient who might fully recover with medical treatment is to cause harm not benefit. Bridge to recovery cannot be assessed without a clinical trial.

The results of cardiac transplantation have improved over the years, partly because of better surgical techniques, greater skill on the part of the surgeon, and the use of modern immunosuppression. But there is another factor, namely the selection of patients for transplantation. In recent years there has been an increasing tendency not to put forward patients who have important renal

dysfunction or evidence of early liver abnormalities. A healthier group of patients is being selected for transplantation and inevitably the results of transplantation have improved. Analysis of outcomes, using statistical methods to adjust for severity of heart failure, is not sufficiently developed to exclude this possibility. Some would argue that in such patients using a device to augment the function of the heart allows time for recovery of renal and hepatic function and that eventually the results of transplantation are improved. That may or may not be so and has yet to be proved in formal scientifically based clinical trials; it is critical that patients in such trials are randomized to the two strategies. But behind that thinking is a weakness of medical judgment. It would be preferable if the judgment to proceed directly to transplantation had been made earlier in such patients so that the argument is really about the timing of transplantation, a failure of proper medical management and strategy.

An alternative argument is that bridge to transplantation allows the possibility that the patient may recover and not require transplantation. But then that is bridge to recovery wrongly diagnosed when the device was inserted. In any event, bridge to recovery seems to be a rare event unless known recoverable conditions, such as myocarditis or alcoholic cardiomyopathy, are present. It is difficult, if not impossible, to understand how longstanding heart failure attributable to a genetic defect can recover spontaneously.

Clinical trials and evidence

The REMATCH trial [2] stands as a monumental achievement in this area of medical care. For the first time a randomized clinical trial was undertaken to evaluate an LVAD device. The device chosen (the HeartMate-1) was rather old fashioned by modern standards. The serious problems with bleeding and infection could easily have been anticipated. Although benefit was demonstrated the effect was small and associated with considerable morbidity. But what this study does underline is that trials can be undertaken and that there is a need for careful clinical trials of new devices, such as the more modern LVADs, in patients who have severe heart failure. Such research is likely to be cost effective [4]. Often physicians and surgeons are reluctant to put patients into such trials because either they believe they are correct in taking a particular course of clinical action or because the ethics and human dilemma of discussing such interventions with patients is too complex. In the view of this writer there is equipoise in undertaking clinical trials because it is equally as unethical to encourage patients to undergo a procedure of unknown benefit as it is to deny patients the advantage of new advances in medical care.

Summary

The idea that patients who have dilated cardiomyopathy (presumably a large heart with near-normal coronary arteries) must have a trial of bridge to recovery is risible. Many such patients should be managed so that they go directly to transplantation and others may be better treated with drug therapy. Some may be more suited to destination therapy. Such a proposal would be immensely costly and is not supported by clear clinical evidence; there has been no trial testing this strategy. Rather, what is needed in this field is more precise terminology, clearer statements of clinical intent at the time of device insertion, improved characterization of patients, more accurate clinical assessment, and above all more information from randomized clinical trials. The failure to undertake and plan such trials, with the exception of the REMATCH study, needs an explanation. The precise reasons for choosing a therapeutic strategy in a patient who has severe heart failure are often obscure and confused.

References

[1] Westaby S, Banning AP, Jarvik R, et al. First permanent implant of the Jarvik 2000 Heart. Lancet 2000; 356:900–3.

[2] Rose EA, Moskowitz AJ, Packer M, et al. The REMATCH trial: rationale, design, and end points. Randomized evaluation of mechanical assistance for the treatment of congestive heart failure. Ann Thorac Surg 1999;67:723–30.

[3] Siegenthaler MP, Westaby S, Frazier OH, et al. Advanced heart failure: feasibility study of long-term continuous axial flow pump support. Eur Heart J 2005;26:1031–8.

[4] Girling AJ, Freeman G, Gordon J, et al. Modelling payback from research into the efficacy of left-ventricular assist devices as destination therapy. Int J Technol Assess Health Care 2007;23(2):269–77.

ELSEVIER
SAUNDERS

Heart Failure Clin 3 (2007) 321–347

HEART
FAILURE
CLINICS

Cardiac Transplantation: Any Role Left?

Martin Cadeiras, MD, Manuel Prinz von Bayern, PhD,
Mario C. Deng, MD, FACC, FESC*

College of Physicians and Surgeons, Columbia University, New York, NY, USA

Heart transplantation was introduced as a breakthrough therapy that dramatically prolonged life in individually selected patients thought to be near death. Unlike most other therapeutic modalities, the survival benefit of cardiac transplantation compared with conventional treatment in advanced heart failure has never been tested in a prospective randomized trial, probably because the benefit of cardiac transplantation compared with conventional therapy usually was assumed clinically evident. The early experience at Stanford University Medical Center between January 1968 and August 1976 demonstrated overall 1- and 2-year survival rates of 52% and 43%, respectively, and a 90% return to functional class I New York Heart Association (NYHA) functional status among transplant survivors, most of them returning to their preillness activities. In this initial series, 95% of the patients selected for transplantation for whom donors did not become available were dead 6 months after evaluation. These data suggested that cardiac transplantation probably not only prolonged survival, but could also return carefully selected recipients to active lives [1]. In 1993, the 24th Bethesda Conference on Cardiac Transplantation recommended heart transplantation as the gold standard therapy in selected patients who had refractory advanced heart failure [2]. Ten years later, according to the established Registry of the International Society for Heart and Lung Transplantation, more than 3000 new transplant patients were being reported to the database each year accounting for a total of 71,040 heart transplants since it started in 1982 [3]. The early observations of the Stanford group may not apply today, because major changes on the understanding and refinement of the therapeutic orchestra available for patients in the advanced phase of heart failure have occurred, specifically with the introduction of highly specialized heart failure units and comprehensive multidisciplinary teams; new pharmacologic compounds, including angiotensin-converting enzyme (ACE) inhibitors, angiotensin-receptor blockers, spironolactone and beta-blockers; novel devices, including trichamber pacemakers, defibrillators, and mechanical circulatory support devices; and improved outcomes with high-risk cardiac surgical procedures. Important improvements in the evaluation of heart transplant patients were achieved after the introduction of functional capacity evaluation by measuring oxygen consumption [4] and subsequently a multivariate model to identify patients at highest risk of death. The heart failure survival score was derived from a prospective cohort and independently validated allowing to dissect the referred population into three groups with low-, medium-, or high-risk profile [5]. Using this tool, a highly provocative national cohort study suggested that heart transplantation may not confer a survival benefit during the first year posttransplantation for patients having low- or medium-risk profiles [6,7]. These findings were supported by subsequent reports using United Network for Organ Sharing

This work was supported at least in part by Grant N HL 077096-01 from the National Institute of Health (MPB, MCD) and by research Funds, Columbia University, Division of Cardiology (MC).

* Corresponding author. Department of Medicine, Division of Cardiology, College of Physicians & Surgeons, Columbia University, 622 West 168th Street, PH12 STEM Room 134, New York NY 10032.

E-mail address: md785@columbia.edu (M.C. Deng).

(UNOS)/Organ Procurement and Transplantation Network (OPTN) data [8–10]. In contrast, the Registry of the International Society of Heart and Lung Transplantation (ISHLT) and the UNOS/OPTN database showed significant improvements in outcomes comparing consecutive eras (1982–1988, 1989–1993, 1994–1998, 1999–2004) achieving a net improvement in median survival from 8.1 to 10.2 years [3]. After the introduction of mechanical circulatory support device (MCSD) in the early 1980s, the Randomized Evaluation of Mechanical Assistance in Treatment of Chronic Heart Failure (REMATCH) study demonstrated a net benefit of mechanical circulatory support for patients who are not eligible for heart transplantation in an extremely sick cohort (NYHA class IV) refractory to conventional medical treatment [11]. Patients in the optimal medical management arm had a 6-month (1 year) mortality of 75 (92)%, whereas in patients randomized to MCSD, the mortality rate was reduced to 52 (25)%. The results of this landmark trial of destination MCSD HeartMate I mechanical assist device (HeartMate, Thoratec, California) led to approval by the US Food and Drug Administration, initiating the era of destination MCSD in the United States. However, this therapy is still far from providing the expected benefits and will require "several miles" of time and effort for this to be achieved as documented in the 3rd Official MCSD—Report of the International Society for Heart and Lung Transplantation [7]. The US Interagency Registry for Mechanical Circulatory Support-National Institutes of Health (NIH) Registry (INTERMACS) constitutes the first obligatory reporting system for patients undergoing destination MCSD implantation.

In this context, the authors aim to analyze the question whether heart transplantation still has a role in the current era of complex technologies. To achieve this objective, the authors first discuss the known benefits of the different therapeutic modalities currently available for patients who have end-stage heart failure, including pharmacologic management, electrophysiologic therapies, high-risk surgical strategies, implantation of mechanical circulatory support device therapy, and heart transplantation. The authors then evaluate the current developments and future perspectives in the field that may influence the likelihood of heart transplantation to remain the therapeutic modality of choice for end-stage heart failure.

Role of pharmacologic treatment in patients who have advanced heart failure

To better assess the current role of orthotopic heart transplantation, we need to start asking ourselves which is the current benefit that medical treatments will add in the medical management of end-stage heart failure. The first randomized prospective clinical trial demonstrating a survival benefit from a medical treatment in advanced heart failure was the CONSENSUS I trial [12]. This study included 256 patients in NYHA IV heart failure and randomized them either to enalapril or placebo. Enalapril conferred a 40% reduction in overall mortality at 6 months, 31% at 1 year, and 27% at the end of study. The mortality rate in the placebo group was 64%, and 46% in the enalapril group. At 10-year follow up, 5 patients, all in the enalapril group, were long-term survivors ($P = .004$). This study is unique in being the first heart failure trial in unselected NYHA IV patients but also in examining extended survival [13]. Increased evidence toward the effects of ACE inhibitors was provided by the Vasodilator–Heart Failure Trial (V-Heft) [14], Studies of Left Ventricular Dysfunction [15], and AIRE [16] studies. The wide availability and rapidly spread use of ACE inhibitors lead to dramatic improvement in the outcomes of these patients. Most challenging was the introduction of betablockers, which were hardly accepted by the scientific community because of their negative chronotropic and lusotropic effect. The effect of blocking the adrenergic system was first attempted two decades before their benefit was tested in a large-scale randomized clinical trial in 7 patients who had advanced congestive cardiomyopathy who had tachycardia at rest. The patients received beta-adrenergic receptor blockade (alprenolol or practolol) for an average 4 to 5 months while in a steady state or progressively deteriorating at the start of beta-adrenergic receptor blockade, on conventional treatment with digitalis and diuretics. Beta-adrenergic blockade improved heart failure clinical symptoms shortly after administration while continued treatment resulted in an increase in physical working capacity and a reduction of heart size. Noninvasive evaluation with phonocardiogram, carotid pulse curve, apex cardiogram, and echocardiogram showed improved ventricular function in all 7 cases. This report suggested that increased catecholamine activity may be an important factor for the development of this disease and of a potential beneficial effect for adrenergic beta-blocking agents [17]. More than 20 years later, the US Carvedilol trial showed a potential benefit for this therapy in patients who had NYHA II and III heart failure. Patients treated with diuretics, digoxin, and ACE inhibitors, mild, moderate, or severe heart failure and left ventricular ejection fractions 35% or less were randomly assigned to receive either placebo (n = 398) or carvedilol (n = 696). The overall mortality rate was 7.8% in the placebo group and 3.2% in the carvedilol group; the reduction in risk attributable to carvedilol was 65% ($P < .001$). This finding led to the termination of the study before its scheduled completion. Carvedilol therapy was also accompanied by a 27% reduction in the risk of hospitalization for cardiovascular causes (19.6% versus 14.1%, $P = .036$), as well as a 38% reduction in the combined risk of hospitalization or death (24.6% versus, 15.8%, $P < .001$) [18]. The efficacy of bisoprolol, a beta-1 selective adrenoceptor blocker, in decreasing all-cause mortality in chronic heart failure was tested in a multicenter double-blind randomized placebo-controlled trial in Europe, the Cardiac Insufficiency Bisoprolol Study-II trial, which evaluated 2647 symptomatic patients in NYHA class III or IV, with left-ventricular ejection fraction of 35% or less receiving standard therapy with diuretics and inhibitors of ACE. Cardiac Insufficiency Bisoprolol Study-II was stopped early, because bisoprolol showed a significant mortality benefit after a mean follow-up of 1.3 years. All-cause mortality and sudden death were significantly lower with bisoprolol than placebo (11.8% versus 17.3%; $P < .0001$, and 3.6% versus 6.3%; $P = .0011$). Treatment effects were independent of the severity or cause of heart failure [19]. The Metoprolol CR/XL Randomized Intervention Trial (MERIT) Study group enrolled 3991 patients who had chronic heart failure in NYHA functional class II to IV and ejection fraction 0.40% or less, stabilized with optimum standard therapy, in a double-blind randomized controlled study. This study randomized 1998 patients to metoprolol CR/XL starting at 12.5 mg (NYHA III–IV) or 25.0 mg once daily (NYHA II) with a target dose of 200 mg once daily uptitrated over 8 weeks, and 2001 patients to placebo. The primary endpoint was all-cause mortality, analyzed by intention to treat. The study was stopped early on the recommendation of the independent safety committee after a mean follow-up of 1 year. All-cause mortality was lower in the metoprolol CR/XL group than in the placebo group (7.2% versus 11.0% per patient-year of follow-up; $P = .0062$). There were fewer sudden deaths and deaths from worsening heart failure in the metoprolol CR/XL group than in the placebo group [20]. The Carvedilol Prospective Randomized Cumulative Survival Study (COPERNICUS) enrolled 2289 patients and demonstrated beneficial effects of therapy with carvedilol on mortality in patients who have NYHA IV chronic heart failure. The placebo 1-year mortality rate of 19.6% was reduced to 11% by carvedilol reflecting a 35% decrease in the risk of death ($P = .0014$). All subgroups including those with the most advanced heart failure showed the same beneficial direction of effect [21]. Based on the results of the studies with carvedilol and metoprolol, a randomized study was designed to randomly evaluate which of these two agents had the greatest efficacy. The Carvedilol or Metoprolol European Trial (COMET) was a multicenter, double-blind, parallel group trial that assigned 1511 patients who had chronic heart failure to treatment with carvedilol (target dose 25 mg twice daily) and 1518 to metoprolol (metoprolol tartrate, target dose 50 mg twice daily). Patients were required to have chronic heart failure (NYHA II-IV), previous admission for a cardiovascular reason, ejection fraction less than 35%, and to have been treated optimally with diuretics and ACE inhibitors unless not tolerated. The mean ejection fraction was 26 ± 7%, and patients were followed during a mean 58 ± 6 months. All-cause mortality was 34% for carvedilol and 40% for metoprolol ($P = .0017$), which was consistent across the predefined subgroups [22].

The use of aldosterone antagonists was first evaluated by the Randomized Aldactone Evaluation Study, which randomized 1663 patients who had severe heart failure (NYHA III and IV) and left ventricular ejection fraction (LVEF) less than 35% treated with angiotensin-converting-enzyme inhibitor, to receive 25 mg of spironolactone daily or placebo. After a mean follow-up period of 24 months, 46% of the patients died in the placebo group and 35% ($P < .001$) in the spironolactone group conferring a 24% reduction in overall mortality at 2 years. This study attributed to reduction of death due to heart failure and of sudden death [23]. Similarly, the use of eplerenone in the Eplerenone Postacute Myocardial Infarction Heart Failure Efficacy and Survival Study (EPHESUS) showed to reduce the incidence of overall mortality and sudden death in patients having acute myocardial infarction that developed heart failure

[24]. A retrospectively analysis in the subgroup of 2106 patients in this trial with LVEF 30% or less showed a 21% relative risk reduction in all-cause mortality ($P = .012$) and 23% for cardiovascular mortality ($P = .008$). The relative risk of sudden cardiac death was reduced 33% ($P = .01$) and heart failure mortality or hospitalization was reduced 25% ($P = .005$). Treatment with eplerenone plus standard therapy in patients who have postacute myocardial infarction heart failure and LVEF 30% or less provided significant incremental benefits in reducing early and late morbidity and mortality [25].

The use of angiotensin receptor blockers was evaluated both as an alternative and in addition to conventional medical treatment in patients who have advanced heart failure. The angiotensin-II type 1 receptor blocker valsartan significantly reduced the combined endpoint of morbidity and mortality and improved clinical signs and symptoms in patients who have heart failure. However, the post hoc observation of an adverse effect on mortality and morbidity in the subgroup receiving valsartan, an ACE inhibitor, and a beta-blocker raised concern about the potential safety of this specific combination [26]. The combined Candesartan in Heart Failure Assessment of Reduction in Mortality and morbidity (CHARM) low LVEF trials, randomized 4576 patients diagnosed of heart failure in NYHA II through IV with a LVEF 40% or less to candesartan (2289 patients) or placebo (2287 patients) in two complementary parallel trials (CHARM-Alternative, for patients who cannot tolerate ACE inhibitors, and CHARM-Added, for patients who were receiving ACE inhibitors). After a median follow-up of 40 months, fewer patients in the Candesartan group experienced cardiovascular death or hospitalization for heart failure compared with the placebo group (37.5% versus. 41.3%), cardiovascular deaths (22.8% versus 26.2%), congestive heart failure (CHF) hospitalizations (22.5% versus 28.1%), and all-cause mortality (28.0% versus 31.0%) [27,28].

The use of positive inotropes/vasodilators treatment using positive inotropes, such as vesnarinone [29,30], xamoterol [31], ibopamine [32], and milrinone [33,34], or vasodilators, such as epoprostenol, did not demonstrate a survival benefit, and, in fact, showed an adverse mortality effect [35]. However, most recent evidence in a limited set of patients indicated that the use of this type of drug, specifically dobutamine and milrinone when combined with an automatic

implantable cardioverter–defibrillator (AICD), is a safe alternative for patients awaiting cardiac transplantation. This strategy may be an acceptable alternative to prolonged hospitalization for patients dependent on continuous inotropic support [36,37]. Phase II results of oral enoximone therapy in intravenous inotrope-dependent subjects demonstrated potential benefit of treatment with this drug [38]. However, the phase III Studies of Oral Enoximone Therapy in Advanced Heart Failure (ESSENTIAL) trials demonstrated a lack of statistically significant differences in all predefined endpoints. Time to all-cause mortality and time to first cardiovascular hospitalization were similar in the enoximone and placebo study groups (21.7% and 22.6%, $P = .73$; 49.4% and 50.1%, $P = .71$, respectively). All-cause mortality and mortality or cardiovascular hospitalization rates were lower with enoximone in the last one half of follow-up (beyond 16.4 months) (5.4% with enoximone versus 8.8% with placebo, $P = .045$; and 12.5% with enoximone versus 17.4% with placebo; $P = .09$). Patients who have LVEF less than 20% had greater improvement in 6-minute walking test distance in the enoximone group [27,39]. Two prospective trials, the "Survival in Patients with Acute Heart Failure in Need of Intravenous Inotropic Support (SURVIVE)" and the "Second Randomized Multicenter Evaluation of Intravenous Levosimendan Efficacy Versus Survival in the Short Term Treatment of Decompensated Heart Failure (REVIVE-II)" could not confirm a substantial benefit of this drug in patients who had advanced heart failure. In the REVIVE-II study, levosimendan was reported to have a superior effect on the composite primary outcome compared with placebo; however, in SURVIVE, despite a trend to early benefit with levosimendan, there was no difference in effect on long-term outcome versus dobutamine [40].

The large number of patients in the most recent trials and the reduced difference in the achieved improvement of outcomes shows the limitation of current interventions to further improve outcomes in patients who have end-stage heart failure [41]. ACE inhibitors, Beta-blockers, and aldosterone receptor blockers remain the cornerstone in the pharmacologic management of heart failure. Any further therapeutic modality should at least show a significant improvement in the benefit conferred by these drugs. Table 1 provides a summary of the major characteristics and outcomes of major clinical trials of pharmacologic intervention.

Table 1
General characteristics and mortality rates of control and treatment arms among major pharmacologic intervention heart failure clinical trials

Study name	Date	Follow up	Total N	NYHA	LVEF	Control	Treatment	Survival benefit
CONSENSUS	1985	6.00	256	4	—	44	26	40.9
V-Heft-I	1986	27.60	642	—	—	34.3	26	24.2
SOLVD Rx	1991	41.40	2569	2–4	31	39.7	35.2	11.3
Vheft-II	1991	24.00	804	2–3	29	25	18	28
U.S. Carvedilol	1996	6.50	1094	2–3	22.5	7.8	3.2	60
ELITE-II	1998	18.00	3152	2–4	31	17.7	15.9	10.2[a]
CIBIS-II	1999	16.00	2647	3–4	27.5	17.3	11.8	31.8
MERIT-HF	1999	12.00	3998	2–4	19	11	7.2	34.5
COPERNICUS	2001	10.40	2289	3–4	19.85	19.6	11	43.8
BEST	2001	24.00	2708	3–4	23.7	33	30	9.1[a]
RALES	2001	24.00	1663	3–4	25	46	35	23.9
CHARM-overall	2003	40.00	4576	2–4	29	31	28	9.7
COMET	2003	58.00	3029	2–4	26	41	35.3	13.9
Val-HEFT	2003	27.00	5010		26.75	19.7	19.4	1.5[a]
ESSENTIAL	2005	6.00	1854	4	25	22.6	21.7	4[a]

Abbreviations: CIBS, Cardiac Insufficiency Bisoprolol Study; COMET, Carvedilol or Metoprolol European Trial; RALES, Randomized Aldactone Evaluation Study; SOLVD, Studies of Left Ventricular Dysfunction.

[a] Nonsignificant.

The American Heart Association (AHA)/ American College of Cardiology (ACC) guidelines for management of heart failure suggest that in patients who have current or prior symptoms of heart failure (stage C) and reduced left ventricular ejection fraction include, among others, the use of angiotensin converting enzyme inhibitors for all patients who have current or prior symptoms of heart failure and reduced LVEF, unless contraindicated, Beta-blockers (using 1 of the 3 proven to reduce mortality [ie, bisoprolol, carvedilol, and sustained release metoprolol succinate]) are recommended for all stable patients who have current or prior symptoms of heart failure (HF) and reduced LVEF, unless contraindicated. Angiotensin II receptor blockers approved for the treatment of HF in patients who have current or prior symptoms of HF and reduced LVEF who are angiotensin–converting enzyme inhibitor–intolerant [42].

Role of electrophysiological treatment in patients who have advanced heart failure

Cardiac resynchronization therapy

The use of implantable devices to resynchronize ventricular contraction may be a beneficial adjunct in the treatment of selected patients who have chronic heart failure. The hypothesis that multisite biventricular pacing may improve myocardial remodeling, hemodynamics, and well-being by reducing ventricular asynchrony, lead to introducing the cardiac resynchronization therapy modality for the management of patients who have advanced heart failure. The Multisite Stimulation in Cardiomyopathies study assessed the clinical efficacy and safety of this new therapy. Sixty-seven patients who had severe heart failure (NYHA III) due to chronic left ventricular systolic dysfunction, with normal sinus rhythm and QRS interval greater than 150 milliseconds, received transvenous atriobiventricular pacemakers. Using a single-blind, randomized, controlled crossover study, it was compared the responses of the patients during two periods: a 3-month period of inactive pacing (ventricular inhibited pacing at a basic rate of 40 bpm) and a 3-month period of active (atriobiventricular) pacing. The mean distance walked in 6 minutes and the quality of life score significantly improved by 22% and 32%, the peak oxygen uptake increased by 8%, and hospitalizations were decreased by two thirds. Active pacing was preferred by 85% of the patients [43]. The Multicenter InSync Randomized Clinical Evaluation (MIRACLE) was the first trial evaluating cardiac resynchronization therapy in a parallel-group randomized evaluation. Patients were in NYHA III or IV heart failure and had a QRS duration of more than 130 milliseconds; 266 patients received a Medtronic InSync device and were then randomized to resynchronization versus no resynchronization for 6 months while background medication was maintained. Patients where defined as "improved" (if they showed improvement in NYHA class or patient global assessment), "unchanged," or "worse" (if they died, had worsening heart failure leading to hospitalization or discontinuation of treatment, or had worse NYHA class or global assessment). Significantly more patients were improved (63% versus 38%) and fewer patients deteriorated (22% versus 29%) in the group with an activated device compared with the control group [44]. The Comparison of Medical Therapy, Pacing, and Defibrillation in Chronic Heart Failure (COMPANION) study, included patients who had NYHA III or IV heart failure, an ejection fraction of 35% or less, and a QRS duration of more than 120 milliseconds. Cardiac-resynchronization therapy with a pacemaker significantly reduced the risk of the combined end point of death from or hospitalization for heart failure by 34%. In patients who had advanced heart failure and a prolonged QRS interval, cardiac-resynchronization therapy decreased the combined risk of death from any cause or first hospitalization while in combination with an implantable defibrillator significantly reduced mortality [45]. In the Cardiac Resyncronization Heart Failure (CARE_HF) study, patients who had NYHA III or IV heart failure due to left ventricular systolic dysfunction and cardiac dyssynchrony who were receiving standard pharmacologic therapy were randomly assigned to receive medical therapy alone or with cardiac resynchronization. A total of 813 patients were enrolled and followed for a mean of 29.4 months. The primary endpoint of time to death from any cause or an unplanned hospitalization for a major cardiovascular event was reached by 39% of the patients in the cardiac-resynchronization group and 55% in the medical-therapy group. All-cause mortality rate was 20% in the cardiac-resynchronization group and 30% in the medical-therapy group [46,47].

Automatic implantable cardiac defibrillator

In the COMPANION study, cardiac-resynchronization therapy with a pacemaker-defibrillator significantly reduced the risk of the combined endpoint of death from or hospitalization for heart failure by 40%. In patients who have advanced heart failure and a prolonged QRS interval, cardiac-resynchronization therapy combined with an implantable defibrillator significantly reduced mortality [45]. The Sudden Cardiac Death in Heart Failure Trial (SCD-HeFT) study compared survival benefit by defibrillator versus amiodarone in 2521 patients who had NYHA II or III heart failure and an ejection fraction of less than 35%. Study groups were conformed by conventional therapy for CHF plus placebo (847 patients), conventional therapy plus amiodarone (845 patients), or conventional therapy plus a conservatively programmed, shock-only, single-lead internal cardio-defibrillator (829 patients). The primary endpoint was death from any cause. The median LVEF was 25%; 70% of the patients were in NYHA II, and 30% were in class III. The etiology of heart failure was ischemic in 52% and nonischemic in 48%. The median follow-up was 45.5 months. Overall mortality was 29% in the placebo group, 28% in the amiodarone group, and 22% in the defibrillator group. Compared with placebo, amiodarone was associated with a similar risk of death, and defibrillator therapy was associated with a 23% significant decrease in the risk of death. Results did not vary according to either ischemic or nonischemic causes of congestive heart failure, but they did vary according to the NYHA class. The authors concluded that in patients who have NYHA II or III CHF and LVEF of 35% or less, amiodarone has no favorable effect on survival, whereas single-lead, shock-only AICD therapy significantly reduces overall mortality [48]. Before SCD-HeFT, the Multicenter Automatic Defibrillator Implantation Trial (MADIT) trial studied whether prophylactic therapy with an implanted cardioverter-defibrillator, compared with conventional medical therapy, would improve survival in a high-risk group of patients who have nonsustained ventricular tachycardia, previous myocardial infarction, and left ventricular dysfunction. Over the course of 5 years, 196 patients in NYHA functional class I to III who had prior myocardial infarction; a left ventricular ejection fraction less than 35%, a documented episode of asymptomatic nonsustained ventricular tachycardia; and inducible, nonsuppressible ventricular tachyarrhythmia on electrophysiologic study were randomly assigned to receive an implanted defibrillator (n = 95) or conventional medical therapy (n = 101). During an average follow-up of 27 months, there was an independent significant reduction of mortality in the defibrillator group compared with the conventional-therapy group [49]. The MADIT II trial demonstrated a 30% all-cause mortality risk reduction from defibrillator implantation in 1232 patients from 76 institutions. The MADIT II was a follow-up study of the MADIT trial. It examined the prophylactic benefit in coronary artery disease patients who had a left ventricular ejection fraction of less than 30%, who have had at least one myocardial infarction but required no further risk stratification. Mean left ventricular ejection fraction was 23.5%, and overall mortality rates were 19.8% and 14.2% in the treatment and control groups, respectively [50]. Table 2 provides a summary of the characteristics and outcomes of major clinical trials of electrophysiologic interventions. The American Heart Association Guidelines for management of patients who have heart failure recommends the use of AICD implantation in patients who have ejection fraction less than 30% and mild to moderate symptoms of HF and in whom survival with good functional capacity is otherwise anticipated to extend beyond 1 year. Because medical therapy may substantially improve ejection fraction, consideration of defibrillator implants should follow documentation of sustained reduction of ejection fraction despite a course of beta-blockers and angiotensin-converting enzyme inhibitors or angiotensin receptor blockers; however, implantable cardiac defibrillators are not warranted in patients who have refractory symptoms of HF (stage D) or in patients who have concomitant diseases that would shorten their life expectancy independent of heart failure [42]. The use of defibrillators and inotropic support in patients who have stage D, class III heart failure was suggested to be a safe and cost-effective alternative for patients in the UNOS status 1B waiting list to be discharged until a suitable donor become identified [36,37].

Role of percutaneous coronary interventions in the management of patients who have advanced heart failure

In the Bypass Angioplasty Revascularization Investigation, patients who had multivessel coronary artery disease were randomly assigned to an initial treatment strategy of coronary artery bypass graft (CABG) (n = 914) or percutaneous transluminal coronary angioplasty (n = 915) and were followed for an average of 5.4 years. Subgroup analysis in a small group of patients who had reduced left ventricular ejection fraction showed 80.7% and 81.1% survival rates in patients undergoing CABG and percutaneous transluminal coronary angioplasty, respectively (83.4% and 89.2% respectively in the group of patients who had diabetes). The observed differences were not statistically significant [51]. The Angina With Extremely Serious Operative Mortality Evaluation (AWESOME) study was a 5-year, multicenter, randomized clinical trial designed to compare long-term survival among patients who had medically refractory myocardial ischemia and high risk of adverse outcomes assigned to either a CABG or a percutaneous coronary intervention (PCI) strategy, which could include stents. Patients from 16 Veterans Affairs Medical Centers were screened to identify myocardial ischemia refractory to medical management and the presence of one or more risk factors for adverse outcome with CABG, including prior open-heart surgery, age over 70 years, left ventricular ejection fraction less than 35%, myocardial infarction within 7 days, or intraaortic balloon pump required. The study included 454 patients consented to random assignment between CABG and PCI. Only 22% of the patients had left ventricular ejection fraction less than 35%, and overall, the mean ejection fraction was less than 45%. The 1-, 6-, and 36-month survival rates for CABG and PCI were 95% versus 97%, 90% versus 94%, and 79% versus 80%, respectively (log-rank test, $P = .46$). Angioplasty was a safe alternative to CABG for patients who had medically refractory myocardial ischemia and high risk of adverse outcomes with CABG [52]. Data from the New York cardiac registries in over

Table 2
General characteristics and mortality rates of control and treatment arms among major electrophysiologic intervention heart failure clinical trials

Study name	Date	Follow-up	Total N	NYHA	LVEF	Control	Treatment	Survival benefit
MIRACLE	2000	6.00	571	3–4	21.7	7.1	5.2	26.8
MADIT-II	2002	20.00	1232	1–4	23.5	19.8	14.2	28.3
COMPANION	2002	12.00	1520	3–4	21.6	19	12	36.8
DEFINITE	2002	24.00	458	1–3	21	14.1	7.9	44
SCD-CHF	2005	45.50	2521	2–3	25	29	22	24.1

Abbreviation: SCD-CHF, sudden cardiac death in heart failure trial.

35,000 patients with multivessel disease who underwent CABG and 20,000 patients who had multivessel disease who underwent PCI from January 1, 1997, to December 31, 2000, was used to determine the rates of death and subsequent revascularization within 3 years after the procedure in various groups of patients according to the number of diseased vessels and the presence or absence of involvement of the left anterior descending coronary artery. The rates of adverse outcomes were adjusted by means of proportional-hazards methods to account for differences in severity of illness before revascularization. Risk-adjusted survival rates were significantly higher among patients who underwent CABG than among those who received a stent in all of the anatomic subgroups studied. In patients who had left ventricular ejection fraction 40% or less, adjusted hazard ratios (95% confidence interval [CI]) for death after CABG compared with stenting (HR = 1.00) by LVEF were as follows: two-vessel, no left anterior descending coronary artery (LAD) disease 0.95 (0.59–1.52); two-vessel, including nonproximal LAD 1.01 (0.67–1.55); two-vessel, including proximal LAD, 0.64 (0.51–0.81); three-vessel, including nonproximal LAD 0.64 (0.48–0.87); and three-vessel, including proximal LAD 0.68 (0.54–0.85). This analysis was based in a registry and therefore should be carefully analyzed. New York State mandates a registry of all patients undergoing PCI and CABG that is monitored by audit and provides survival data on all New York State residents [53]. The ACC/AHA practice guidelines for percutaneous coronary interventions states that is reasonable to perform routine percutaneous coronary interventions in patients who have left ventricular ejection fraction 40% or less, heart failure, and/or serious ventricular arrhythmias although the evidence is limited [54].

Role of surgical treatment in patients who have advanced heart failure

Coronary artery bypass surgery

High-risk revascularization may constitute the treatment of choice in the subgroup of advanced heart failure patients who have ischemic cardiomyopathy, an ejection fraction less than 35%, viable myocardium, and vessels suitable for grafting. The NIH-sponsored Surgical Treatment for Ischemic Heart Failure (STICH) trial includes 2800 patients to evaluate whether surgical

coronary revascularization in addition to aggressive medical heart failure management confer long-term mortality, morbidity, quality of life, or cost benefits beyond aggressive medical management alone in patients who have symptomatic heart failure, left ventricular dysfunction, and coronary artery disease amenable to CABG and whether surgical ventricular shape restoration in combination with CABG improve outcome compared with coronary revascularization alone and medical therapy alone [55]. As of November 2006, 1900 patients have been enrolled [56]. Nonrandomized observations in patients who had left ventricular dysfunction and heart failure from 5410 patients who had ischemic left ventricular dysfunction who were enrolled in the Studies of Left Ventricular Dysfunction trials were retrospectively evaluated. Outcomes of patients who had (n = 1870, 35%) and who did not have (n = 3540, 65%) history of prior CABG were compared and stratified by baseline ejection fraction values (<0.25, 0.25 to 0.30, and >0.30). Prior CABG was associated with a 25% reduction in risk of death and a 46% reduction in risk of sudden death independent of ejection fraction and severity of heart-failure symptoms [57]. Early results of benefit of CABG in 39 patients who had preoperative ejection fractions less than 20% who underwent coronary artery bypass, showed a 3-year survival rate of 83% [58]. Different trials have suggested the benefit of revascularization in advanced heart failure if angina [59] or hibernation [60–65] is present. If no viable myocardium is present, the prospect of improvement with revascularization is reduced and, thus, cardiac transplantation should be considered for appropriate candidates [58,66–68]. Only few studies compared PCI and CABG for high-risk patients who had ischemia and severely compromised ejection fraction. Although a nonrandomized comparison, the New York Registry analysis is among the best currently available evidence favoring surgery over PCI in patients who have ejection fraction 40% or less and severe two-vessel disease including proximal LAD or severe three-vessel disease with and without proximal compromise of the LAD [53].

Mitral valve surgery

The effect of mitral valve surgery on patients who have end-stage heart failure was evaluated in a nonrandomized study by the group at the University of Michigan–Ann Arbor, which studied the intermediate-term outcome of mitral reconstruction in 48 patients who had cardiomyopathy with severe mitral regurgitation (63 ± 6 years, EF 16% ± 3%, maximal drug therapy, NYHA III–IV, refractory 4+ mitral regurgitation). All 48 patients had undersized flexible annuloplasty rings inserted, 7 had coronary bypass grafts for incidental disease, 11 had prior bypass grafts, and 11 also had tricuspid valve repair. One operative death occurred as a result of right ventricular failure. The 1- and 2-year actuarial survivals were 82% and 71%. At a mean follow-up of 22 months, the number of hospitalizations for heart failure has decreased, and 1 patient has had heart transplantation. Significantly, NYHA class improved from 3.9 ± 0.3 before the operation to 2.0 ± 0.6 after the operation. Twenty-four months after the operation, left ventricular volume and sphericity decreased, whereas ejection fraction and cardiac output repeatedly increased [69]. A retrospective analysis of 126 consecutive patients, who had significant mitral regurgitation and left ventricular systolic dysfunction on echocardiography, undergoing mitral valve annuloplasty between 1995 and 2002, did not demonstrate a clear survival benefit [70]. The Acorn study prospectively evaluated the safety and efficacy of mitral valve surgery with and without the CorCap cardiac support device (Acorn Cardiovascular, St. Paul, Minnesota) in patients who had NYHA II to IV heart failure. A subgroup of 193 patients were enrolled in the mitral valve repair or replacement stratum of the Acorn Clinical Trial; 102 patients were randomized to the mitral valve surgery alone group (control), and 91 patients were randomized to mitral valve surgery with implantation of the CorCap cardiac support device. Patients were followed for a median duration of 22.9 months. For the entire mitral valve surgery group, the 30-day operative mortality rate was 1.6%. Mitral surgery was associated with progressive reductions in left ventricle end-diastolic volume, left ventricle end-systolic volume and left ventricular mass, and increases in left ventricle ejection fraction and sphericity index. Recurrence of clinically significant mitral regurgitation was uncommon. Quality of life, exercise performance, and NYHA functional class were all improved [71]. Currently, the recommendations of the AHA for management of patients who have valvular heart disease states that mitral valve surgery is reasonable for patients who have chronic,

nonischemic, severe mitral regurgitation due to a primary abnormality of the mitral apparatus NYHA functional class III or IV and severe left ventricular dysfunction defined as ejection fraction less than 30% and/or end-systolic dimension greater than 55 mm in whom mitral valve repair is highly likely. Level of evidence is limited to consensus opinion of experts, case studies, or standard of care as it is for patients who have chronic severe secondary mitral regurgitation due to severe left ventricular dysfunction who have persistent NYHA functional class III or IV symptoms despite optimal therapy for heart failure including biventricular pacing. In these patients, mitral valve repair may be considered [72].

Aortic valve surgery

Whether aortic valve surgery among patients who have severe aortic valvular disease or severe left ventricular dysfunction is associated with improved survival in comparison to medical treatment or transplantation has not been widely studied. The outcome of aortic valve replacement in patients who have severe aortic stenosis, low transvalvular gradient, and severe left ventricular dysfunction was evaluated in 52 patients with mean ejection fraction, 26 ± 8%; aortic valve mean gradient, 23 ± 4 mmHg; aortic valve area, 0.7 ± 0.2 cm^2; and cardiac output, 3.7 ± 1.2 L/min. Simultaneous coronary artery bypass graft surgery was performed in 32 patients (62%). Total mortality in this series was 40%. The multivariate analysis showed smaller prosthesis size as the only predictor of surgical mortality. Postoperative functional improvement occurred in most patients, and postoperative ejection fraction improved in 74% of the patients evaluated. Despite severe left ventricular dysfunction, low transvalvular mean gradient, and increased operative mortality, aortic valve replacement was associated with improved functional status. Postoperative survival was related to younger patient age and larger aortic prosthesis size, and medium-term survival was related to improved postoperative functional class [73]. Another single center experience evaluated 68 patients between 1990 and 1998 that underwent aortic valve replacement for severe aortic stenosis with low valvular gradient, and 89 patients who did not undergo aortic valve replacement with an aortic valve area 0.75 cm^2 or less, left ventricular ejection fraction 35% or less, and mean gradient 30 mm Hg or less. Survival was compared between a cohort of

39 patients in the aortic valve replacement group and 56 patients in the control group. One- and 4-year survival rates were markedly improved in patients in the aortic valve replacement group (82% and 78%) compared with patients in the control group (41% and 15%; $P < .0001$). By multivariable analysis, the main predictor of improved survival was aortic valve replacement [74]. Perioperative outcomes and long-term results were also evaluated in a group of 132 consecutive patients who had impaired left ventricular systolic function ($<40\%$) undergoing aortic valve replacement with or without concomitant CABG between 1990 and 2003. Patients who had other valve pathology were excluded. Preoperatively, 82% of the patients were in NYHA III or IV. Sixty patients (45%) underwent aortic valve replacement for severe aortic stenosis, whereas 72 (55%) had aortic insufficiency. In the aortic stenosis group, the mean left ventricular ejection fraction and aortic valve area were $26 \pm 4\%$ and 0.8 ± 0.4 cm^2, respectively. All patients had a mean LVEF of $27 \pm 6\%$ and a mean left ventricular end-systolic diameter of 52 ± 9 mm. Fifty-seven (43%) required concomitant CABG. LVEF increased to $29 \pm 10\%$ and $34 \pm 12\%$ after 6 months in the aortic stenosis and aortic insufficiency groups, respectively. The mean follow-up period was 6.1 years with no differences for both groups with respect to either perioperative or long-term outcomes. Overall survival was 96%, 79%, and 55% at 1, 5, and 10 years, respectively [75]. Overall, these results suggests that both aortic valve replacement for patients who have low gradient aortic stenosis and aortic regurgitation confines a greater survival benefit than that of heart transplantation, although special care should be taken in the selection of prosthetic valve used for replacement. The ACC/AHA guidelines for evaluation of patients who have aortic valve disease states that aortic valve replacement is indicated for symptomatic patients who have severe aortic regurgitation irrespective of left ventricular systolic function as well as in patients who have severe aortic stenosis and left ventricular systolic dysfunction, which is defined as ejection fraction less than 50% [72].

Left ventricular geometry restoration

Prospective randomized comparison is being conducted by the STICH trial, which evaluates whether surgical ventricular shape restoration in combination with CABG improve outcome compared with coronary revascularization alone and medical therapy alone in one of the study arms [56]. The safety and efficacy of surgical anterior ventricular endocardial restoration, which includes the exclusion of noncontracting segments in the dilated remodeled ventricle after anterior myocardial infarction was evaluated in an observational effort of 11 centers. From January 1998 to July 1999, 439 patients underwent the procedure and were followed for 18 months. Concomitant with safety and efficacy of surgical anterior ventricular endocardial restoration, coronary artery bypass grafting was done in 89% of the patients, mitral valve repair in 22%, and replacement in 4%. Hospital mortality was 6.6%. Postoperatively, ejection fraction increased from 29 ± 10.4 to $39 \pm 12.4\%$, and left ventricular end-systolic volume index decreased from 109 ± 71 to 69 ± 42 mL/m^2 ($P < .005$). At 18 months, survival was 89.2% (84% in the overall group and 88% among the 421 patients who had coronary artery bypass grafting or mitral valve repair) [76]. The international Reconstructive Endoventricular Surgery returning Torsion Original Radius Elliptical shape to the left ventricle (RESTORE) group evaluated surgical ventricular restoration in a registry of 1198 postinfarction patients between 1998 and 2003. Concomitant procedures included CABG in 95%, mitral valve repair in 22%, and mitral valve replacement in 1%. Overall 30-day mortality was 5.3% (8.7% with mitral repair versus 4.0% without repair, $P < .001$). Perioperative mechanical support was uncommon ($<9\%$). Left ventricular ejection fraction increased from $29.6 \pm 11.0\%$ to $39.5 \pm 12.3\%$ ($P < .001$), and left ventricular end systolic volume index decreased from 80.4 ± 51.4 mL/m^2 to 56.6 ± 34.3 mL/m^2 ($P < .001$). Overall 5-year survival was $68.6 \pm 2.8\%$. In this study, and ejection fraction 30% or less, left ventricular end-systolic volume 80 mL/m^2 or greater, advanced NYHA functional class, and age equal or greater than 75 years as risk factors for death. Five-year freedom from hospital readmission for CHF was 78%. Preoperatively, 67% of patients were class III or IV, and postoperatively 85% were class I or II. Based on these data, the authors concluded that surgical ventricular restoration improves ventricular function and is highly effective therapy in the treatment of ischemic cardiomyopathy with excellent 5-year outcome [76]. The results of the STICH trial will probably solve the real role of surgical restoration therapy compared with conventional approaches.

Role of mechanical circulatory support as a destination therapy in the treatment of patients who have advanced heart failure

Destination mechanical circulatory support therapy has become an option for end-stage heart failure patients not eligible for heart transplantation in whom all lifestyle and medical options have been exhausted without success, in the setting of decompensation and progression of advanced heart failure, a phase known to be associated with a high risk of death. The RE-MATCH trial, established for the first time in the mechanical circulatory support field, a survival benefit and quality of life benefit from MCSD implantation [11] in patients who have end-stage heart failure who are ineligible for cardiac transplantation, showed a 48% reduction in the risk of death from any cause in the group randomly assigned to MCSD compared with those under optimal medical management. MCSD patients had a significantly greater chance of suffering serious adverse events but provided a significant improvement in quality of life. A recent analysis of the REMATCH cohort supported the initial observation beyond 2 years. As of July 2003, 11 patients were alive on MCSD support of a total 16 survivors, including 3 crossover patients originally receiving optimal medical management. This analysis also showed a significant improvement in survival for MCSD supported patients enrolled during the second half of the trial compared with the first half [77]. Patients requiring inotropic support in this study population at the time of MCSD implantation showed the highest likelihood of benefit in terms of survival and improved quality of life, whereas patients not undergoing inotropic infusions had a tendency to higher survival rates both with and without MCSD [78], implying that only in patients who are inotrope-dependent are therefore likely to have a 1-year survival probability without MCSD implantation of less than 50%; MCSD intervention will add to survival and quality of life benefit. A retrospective analysis including 255 recipients of the Novacor assist device (Rueil-Malmaison, Cedex, France) showed comparable effects as the HeartMate I device (Thoratec, Pleasanton, California) [79]. Second-generation permanent axial flow devices may also evolve as a treatment option in ineligible and selected elderly patients who have end-stage heart failure [80,81]. According to the third annual ISHLT-MCSD report, the vast majority of patients are triaged to destination MCSD because of advanced age or severe comorbidities that make them poorly suited for transplantation. Most of these patients received pulsatile MCSDs. Among the entire cohort of destination patients, the actuarial survival was 65% at 6 months and 34% at 1 year. As shown in the multivariable analysis for the overall group, older age remains a major risk factor for mortality. Among patients less than 65 years of age at the time of destination therapy, the actuarial survival at 1 year was 41%, and for those over the age of 65, it was less than 30% [7]. Complications of long-term mechanical circulatory support include infections, coagulopathies, right ventricular failure, arrhythmias, and device dysfunction. Infection causes substantial morbidity and mortality after MCSD implantation and reduces the survival and quality-of-life benefit [82–84]. The third MCSD report demonstrates that infection continues to be the major complication limiting outcomes at 1 year [7]. Next to infection, coagulation problems leading to clotting stroke limited the survival and quality of life benefit from long-term mechanical support in the REMATCH experience [85]. As opposed to the risk of infection, which augments linearly after MCSD implantation, the risk of coagulopathies including bleeding and clot-associated embolic stroke is clustered in the early postoperative period. At the time of decision making, high-risk subgroups to consider include concurrent placement of right ventricular assist device (RVAD), older age, female gender, lower platelet count, higher white blood cell count, blood type A, diabetes, preimplant ventilator, and higher creatinine values [7]. Although MCSD pumping leads to a progressive decrease in pulmonary vascular resistance and normalization of pulmonary pressures, improving right ventricular performance and geometry [86,87] insertion of an implantable MCSD complicated by early right ventricular failure has a poor prognosis [7]. Device dysfunction can complicate the follow-up. Within established types of MCSDs, improvements have been made to ensure better outcomes [87]. In a single-center report, the cumulative probability of device failure gradually increased up to 64% at 2 years [88]. Table 3 provides a summary of the characteristics and outcomes of major experiences of mechanical circulatory support as destination therapy. Recently the ISHLT published guidelines for evaluation and selection of patients undergoing MCSD implantation [89].

Table 3
General characteristics and survival rates of control and treatment arms among major mechanical circulatory support device intervention heart-failure studies

Study name	References	Total N	6 Mo	12 Mo	24 Mo
DW Heart Center	Jurman [80]	27	32	22	22
Jarvik 2000	Siegenthaler [81]	17		56	47
REMATCH	Park [Park, 2001]	129	60	52	29
ISHLT DT 2nd Report	Deng [7]	35	65	34	
ISHLT 2nd Report	Deng [7]	413	68	55	

Data from Cadeiras M, Von Bayern MP, Pal A, et al. Destination therapy: an alternative for end-stage heart failure patients not eligible for heart transplantation. Curr Opin Organ Transplant 2005;10:369–75.

Role of heart transplantation in patients who have advanced heart failure

During the past 2 decades, improved outcomes with medical and surgical therapy and different trends in cardiac transplantation have reduced the comparative survival benefit gained with cardiac transplantation in certain populations when compared with conventional therapy. The death rates of patients on the UNOS (www.unos.org) waiting list (depicted as deaths per 1000 patient years spent on the waiting list) have decreased dramatically over time (Table 4), from 432.2 in 1990 to 198.1 in 1999 and 156.2 in 2004. The death rate in 2004 was the lowest of the past 15 years. However, registrants in the most medically urgent status category (UNOS status 1A) had much higher death rates than did others. The death rate for status 1A registrants in 2004 was 547.7 compared with 332.5 for status 1B and 96.9 for status 2 registrants. In comparison with waiting list outcomes, for the 2001 to 2004 cardiac transplantation cohort, the 1-year survival rate in the United States was 86.7%. Recipients in medical urgency status 1 at the time of transplantation had slightly lower 1-year survival rates than recipients in status 2 at the time of transplantation (86.5% versus 90.6%) (UNOS database, queried November 11, 2006). Because annualized mortality rates per 1000 patient years at risk and Kaplan-Meier depictions of survival cannot be compared directly, an estimate of the survival benefit with cardiac transplantation in the UNOS status 1 versus status 2 groups is not possible. The ISHLT Registry (www.ishlt.org) indicates an improvement of 1-year survival after cardiac transplantation from 80.5% between 1989 and 1993 to 82.18% between 1994 and 1998 and 84.89 between 1999 and 2004. It does not provide data on waiting list mortality [3]. In a prospective observational cohort study, all 889 adult patients listed for a first heart transplant in Germany in 1997 were followed up to assess mortality and stratified by heart failure severity. Within 1 year after listing, patients who had a predicted high risk had the highest global death rate (51% versus 32% and 29% for medium and low risk patients respectively; $P < .0001$), the highest risk of dying on the waiting list (32% versus 20% and 20%; $P = .0003$), and were more likely to receive a transplant (48% versus 45% and 41%; $P = .01$). Differences between the risk groups in outcome after transplantation did not reach significance ($P = .2$). Transplantation was not associated with a reduction in mortality risk for the total cohort, but it did provide a survival benefit for the high-risk group. Based on these data, the authors concluded that cardiac transplantation in Germany was associated with a survival benefit

Table 4
Survival rates currently reported in United Network for Organ Sharing/Organ Procurement and Transplantation Network International Society for Heart and Lung Transplantation registries in patients in the waiting list stratified by United Network for Organ Sharing status and heart transplant recipients

Registry	Period	12 mo	36 mo	60 mo	Source
Waiting list status 1A	1997–2004	85.7	75.2	68.8	UNOS/OPTN
Waiting list status 1B	1997–2004	87.4	80.2	72.6	UNOS/OPTN
Waiting list status 2	1997–2004	90.6	81.8	74	UNOS/OPTN
Heart transplant	1999–2004	84.9	78.6	72.1	UNOS/ISHLT

only in patients who had a predicted high risk of dying on the waiting list and suggested that patients who had a predicted low or medium risk have no reduction in mortality risk associated with transplantation, and therefore, they should be managed with organ-saving approaches rather than transplantation [6]. This hypothesis was supported by two other retrospective analyses that used data from the UNOS database on 7539 adult patients that were listed for transplantation between January 1999 and June 2001. Of these, 4255 (56.4%) patients were listed as UNOS status 2. Final outcomes on the waiting list for patients initially listed as UNOS status 2 were transplantation (48%), removal from the list (11.5%), death (11.4%), and continued listing (29%). At 30 months after transplantation, survival was 81% for patients undergoing transplantation as status 1A, 77% as status 1B, and 83% as status 2, and showed no difference among groups. At 365 days, survival analysis showed no difference for patients listed and undergoing transplantation as UNOS status 2 compared with those still waiting as status 2 [10].

Recently, a decision-analytic model was created to simulate a randomized clinical trial of optimal medical therapy versus heart transplantation for each NYHA class by calculating the average life expectancy. Assumptions for annual mortality in the optimal medical treatment group were no excess mortality from heart failure for class I patients, 5.3% and 8.1% for class II and III based on the results of the MERIT-HF study and 12.8% for class IV heart failure based on the COPERNICUS study. Mortality related to heart transplantation was based on UNOS survival curves for the period 1982 to 2001. For classes I, II, and III, optimal medical treatment demonstrated a life expectancy gain of 113 months (232 ± 2.2 versus 119 ± 2.1), 38 months (152 ± 2.1 versus 114 ± 2.1), and 6 months (117 ± 1.8 versus 111 ± 2.2), respectively, over heart transplantation, whereas class IV favored heart transplantation with a life expectancy gain of 26 months (107 ± 2.1 versus 81 ± 1.4) over optimal medical therapy. According to this model, currently, optimal medical treatment is superior to HT for classes I, II, and III, but HT is superior for class IV. However, future advances in optimal medical treatment or HT may change the relative benefits of these treatment modalities [9]. Questions would arise whether the performance of classical tools still identify patients that are too well for transplantation in the modern era of management of

advanced heart failure [90]. The prognostic value of variables used for risk stratification of patients who have congestive heart failure was markedly influenced by beta-blocker treatment [91]. The performance of peak VO_2 and the Heart Failure Survival Score have been reevaluated on 2105 patients referred for cardiopulmonary testing. Peak VO_2 was a predictor of mortality irrespective of beta-blocker use; a decrease of 1 mL x kg(-1) x minute(-1) resulted in an adjusted hazard ratio of 1.13 (95% CI 1.09 to 1.17, $P < .0001$) in patients not receiving beta-blockers and 1.27 (95% CI 1.18 to 1.36, $P < .0001$) in patients receiving beta-blockers [92]. Beta-blocker use was associated with better outcomes until peak VO_2 values became low (approximately 10 mL x kg[-1] x minute[-1]), at which level survival rates were equally poor. Therefore, peak VO_2 remains as a determinant of survival in patients who have heart failure even in the setting of beta-blockade. Because of improved survival in patients treated with beta-blockers, the cut point value of 14 mg x kg(-1) x minute(-1) for referral for cardiac transplantation in these patients required re-evaluation [93]. The likelihood of benefit of transplantation in the current era was evaluated analyzing peak VO_2 and heart failure survival score in 320 patients followed from 1994 to 1997 (past era) and in 187 patients followed from 1999 to 2001 (current era) and comparing outcomes between these two groups of patients and those who underwent heart transplantation from 1993 to 2000. Survival in the past era was 78% at 1 year and 67% at 2 years, compared with 88% and 79%, respectively, in the current era (both $P < .01$). One-year event-free survival (without urgent transplantation or left ventricular assist device) was improved in the current era, regardless of initial peak VO_2: 64% versus 48% for peak VO_2 less than 10 mL/min/kg ($P = .09$), 81% versus 70% for 10 to 14 mL/min/kg ($P = .05$), and 93% versus 82% for >14 mL/min/kg ($P = .04$). Of the patients who had peak VO_2 of 10 to 14 mL/min/kg, 55% had low-risk heart failure survival score and exhibited 88% 1-year event-free survival. One-year survival after transplantation was 88%, which is similar to the 85% rate reported by the UNOS for 1999 to 2000 [8]. To ascertain survival of ischemic advanced heart failure patients by treatment allocation, the assessment outcome of transplant patients allocated to medical therapy, high-risk conventional surgery, or transplantation were identified from the Papworth transplant database and excluded if primary etiology was not ischemic. Grouping was undertaken according to treatment allocation at initial assessment, and analysis was performed by intention to treat. Survival was computed from the time of assessment and Cox regression used to stratify patients according to risk with the Heart Failure Survival Score. From May 1993 to September 2001, a total of 755 patients were admitted for transplant assessment, with 348 (46.1%) identified as having heart failure of ischemic origin. Variables required for calculation of the Heart Failure Survival Score was available in 273 patients (78.4%), and 20 patients (7.3%) were lost to follow-up. Of the remaining 253 patients, 89 (35.2%) were allocated to medical therapy, 32 (12.6%) to surgery, and 132 (52.2%) to transplantation. The relative risk (95% confidence limit) of death compared with medical therapy was 0.62 (0.28, 1.40) for surgery and 0.38 (0.24, 0.61) for transplantation in medium- to high-risk patients. For low-risk patients, the relative risks for death compared with medical therapy were 1.87 (0.63, 5.60) for surgery and 1.97 (0.79, 4.96) for transplantation. Transplantation improved survival of medium- and high-risk patients compared with medical therapy. In the low-risk group, this was not evident. However, repeated assessment of risk is required because the hazard for death rises steadily after the third year in these patients [94].

Cardiac transplantation: any role left?

Whether heart transplantation will still remain a therapeutic option for the future management of advanced heart failure will likely depend on (1) the emergence of new therapies and improvement of current management of end-stage heart failure, and (2) the emergence of new therapies and improvement of current management of heart transplantation. Figs. 1 and 2 depicts mortality rates in patients from different clinical trials in control (see Fig. 1) and intervention (see Fig. 2) groups, combined with reported outcomes by the UNOS/OPTN database stratified by UNOS urgency status and last reported ISHLT transplant database outcomes. Possibilities to improve interventions may require clinicians and basic scientists within the translational research programs to make joint efforts and find new ways for understanding and designing strategies to face the problem of heart failure and transplantation. A recent study combined data from randomized clinical trials and (MERIT and COPERNICUS) and UNOS survival curves to simulate a randomized clinical trial. Sensitivity analysis revealed if improvement in optimal medical therapy decreased mortality by 38% for class IV patients, optimal medical therapy and heart transplantation would have equivalent life expectancies. If improvement in heart transplantation resulted in a 7% increase in postheart-transplantation survival, optimal medical therapy and heart transplantation would be equivalent for class III patients. If improvement in heart transplantation resulted in a 30% increase in postheart-transplantation survival, optimal medical therapy and heart transplantation would be equivalent for class II patients [9].

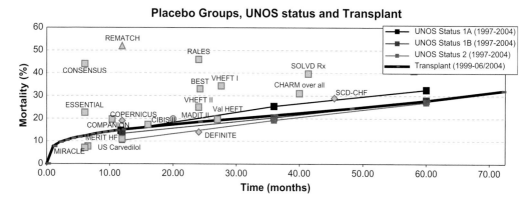

Fig. 1. General comparative analysis of outcomes patients listed for heart transplantation as status 1A, 1B, and 2, patients undergoing Orthotopic Heart Transplantation, and patients in the placebo groups reported by major clinical trials. (*Data from* the OPTN, UNOS/ISHLT database.)

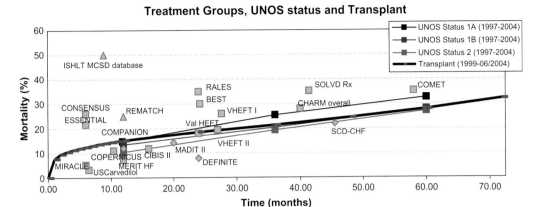

Fig. 2. General comparative analysis of outcomes patients listed for heart transplantation as status 1A, 1B, and 2, patients undergoing Orthotopic Heart Transplantation, MCSD implantation, and patients in the treatment groups reported by major clinical trials. (*Data from* the OPTN, UNOS/ISHLT database.)

Emergence of new therapies and improvement of current management of end-stage heart failure

Improving current management of end stage heart failure

Is it yet possible to improve management of patients being treated with heart failure? An amount of evidence favors the concept that multidisciplinary heart-failure dedicated teams with strong nursing support and educational intervention reduces mortality by improving compliance and preventing decompensation. A global application of this concept still needs to be met. A meta-analysis evaluating the long-term impact of chronic heart-failure management programs to determine whether multidisciplinary strategies improve outcomes for heart failure patients showed that strategies that incorporated follow-up by a specialized multidisciplinary team reduced mortality, hospitalizations for heart failure, and all-cause hospitalizations [95]. A randomized controlled trial that included 223 patients compared the effects of a 1-hour, one-on-one teaching session with a nurse educator to the standard discharge process. Subjects randomized to receive the teaching session had fewer days hospitalized or dead in the follow-up period, lower risk of rehospitalization or death, and lower costs of care [96]. The effects of a nurse-led, multidisciplinary, home-based intervention to usual postdischarge care after a short-term hospitalization was compared for up to 10 years of follow-up in 297 patients. Median survival in the home-based intervention cohort (n = 149) almost doubled that of usual care group and significantly

reduced overall mortality. Home-based intervention was associated with prolonged event-free survival [97,98].

The use of implantable monitoring devices and measuring of internal thoracic impedance may be adopted in the future to help management of patients who have end stage heart failure. The Chronicle Offers Management Patients with Advanced Signs and Symptoms of Heart Failure (COMPASS-HF) study used an implantable device that continuously monitors intracardiac pressures. Patients were randomized to receive optimal heart failure care alone (140 patients) or optimal heart failure care and therapy guided by the Chronicle (Medtronic, Minneapolis, Minnesota) device (134 patients). Implantable monitoring showed to be safe and to improve patients who have NYHA III or IV chronic heart failure [99]. Impedance cardiography uses changes in thoracic electrical impedance to estimate hemodynamic variables. The Prospective Evaluation and Identification of Decompensation by Impedance Cardiography Test study prospectively assessed the potential utility of impedance cardiography assessed by the BioZ ICG Monitor (CardioDynamics, San Diego, California) device in predicting clinical deterioration in 212 ambulatory patients who had heart failure and a recent episode of clinical decompensation. A composite score composed by velocity index, thoracic fluid content index, and left ventricular ejection time assessed by this method was powerful to predict the occurrence of a new event during the following 2 weeks [41]. Ongoing developments include, among others, the Chronicle AICD (Medtronic, Minneapolis, Minnesota) device, which features AICD's capability and real-time intraventricular pressure monitoring, body temperature, patient activity and heart rate permanently. The information is then transmitted to their treating team by way of telephone.

Developing better pharmacologic strategies

Current trends in the identification of new effective pharmacologic targets seem to have reached a plateau. The benefits of incremental and selective neurohormonal blockade in patients who have heart failure might become saturated [100]. Studies with novel compounds that aimed to interfere with the detrimental effects of neurohormones and inflammatory mediators based on monocausal hypotheses failed to provide additional benefit to the current standards of therapy. The endopeptidase inhibitor Omapatrilat was effective in reducing the endpoint of death or hospitalization in patients who had chronic NYHA II to IV heart failure when compared with enalapril, but it was not more effective than this drug alone [101]. Trials with Moxonidine, a central acting agent, blocker of the norepinephrine outflow [102], the endothelin receptor blockers Bosentan [103], Tezosentan [104–106], and Darusentan [107,108], the TNF receptor blockers Etanercept [109–111] and Infliximab [112] failed to show significant survival benefit in the advanced heart failure population. Although novel, the mobilization of bone marrow cells by hematopoietic growth factors was used on the REVIVAL-2 trial, which used a granulocyte-colony stimulating factor to stimulate bone-marrow cells to regenerate cardiac tissue in patients who have acute myocardial infarction. Treatment with granulocyte-colony stimulating factor did not change left ventricular function or reduce infarct size at follow-up [113].

The emergence of stem cells as a *holy-grail* of end-stage heart failure, although revolutionary, its effectiveness still needs to be supported. The Bone Marrow Transfer to enhance ST-elevation infarct regeneration (BOOST) trial was a randomized evaluation in which 60 patients having undergone successful percutaneous coronary intervention for acute ST-segment elevation myocardial infarction received either optimal postinfarction medical treatment (controls) or intracoronary transfer of autologous bone-marrow cells in addition to optimal medical treatment. Bone-marrow cells were inoculated after a mean of 4.8 days after percutaneous coronary intervention. Left ventricular ejection fraction after 6 months as determined by cardiac MRI, increased 0.7% in the control group and 6.7% in the bone-marrow-cell group [114]. In a series of 18 patients that were 5 months to 8.5 years after myocardial infarction, mononuclear cells isolated from the iliac crest bone-marrow were then readministered by way of an intracoronary balloon catheter directly into the infarcted zone. Baseline tests of exercise capacity, ventricular function, coronary stenosis, and infarct size were repeated 3 months after intracoronary infusion of cells. Infarct size was reduced by 30%, while global left ventricular ejection fraction and regional infarct wall-movement velocity improved by 15% and 57%, respectively. Data was contrasted against 18 patients who had chronic myocardial infarction but no stem-cell therapy [115]. The Reinfusion of Enriched Progenitor Cells and Infarct Remodeling in Acute Myocardial Infarction (REPAIR-AMI) study randomized patients to stem cell treatment in patients who had myocardial infarction. Intracoronary infusion of progenitor cells taken from the patient's own bone marrow marginally improved the ejection fraction [116]. The same group reported an average 2.9% improvement in left ventricular ejection fraction among patients receiving bone marrow cells. The increase in global cardiac function was related to significantly enhance of regional contractility in the area targeted by intracoronary infusion of bone marrow cells. The crossover phase of the study revealed a significant increase in global and regional left ventricular function [117]. Although the benefit of cell therapy is still limited, it is yet in an early stage, and future development may lead to better results that will need to be tested in larger scale randomized clinical trials.

The current standard of scientific thought may probably need to be evaluated. Probably, shifting from the monocausal-single mechanism hypothesis/blockade to a systems-biology based approach directed to the understanding of key regulatory pathways that are detrimental and targeting specific compounds regulating these pathways with an ad hoc understanding of the perturbation generated in the whole system. A change from a reductionist paradigm toward the challenge of dealing with complexity may find new roads for development and advancement of heart failure. From a pharmacologic approach, after completion of the human genome project [118], having a comprehensive catalog of all the members of a given gene family in the human genome allows one to take a different perspective on the drug-discovery process [119]. Chemogenomic approaches may allow distinguishing the molecular targets of a bioactive compound from the hundreds to thousands of additional gene products that respond indirectly to changes in the activity of the targets. Integrated computational–experimental approach for computing the likelihood that gene products and associated pathways are targets of a compound can be achieved by filtering the mRNA expression profile of compound-exposed cells using a reverse-engineered model of the cell's gene regulatory network [120,121].

Improving outcomes with current and newer generation assist devices

The improvements of infection management and coagulation protocols are currently being addressed at the Specialized Centers for Clinically Oriented Research (SCCOR) program lead by Columbia University on the biology of human mechanical circulatory support. In this large-scale project, a multicenter effort wants to identify new means of controlling the coagulation cascade to prevent thrombotic events, prevention of assist device infection and myocardial recovery by cardiac unloading and stem cell implantation (NIH-NHLBI HL 077,096-01). Several ongoing efforts include the development of totally implanted pumps with levitating rotary surfaces and transcutaneal energy sources to minimize infection. A special section in this issue of *Heart Failure Clinics* is dedicated to analyzing current possibilities of improving MCSD.

Improving selection of patients undergoing mechanical circulatory support device implantation and identifying those with high likelihood of recovery for Bridge to Recovery strategy

A review on current status of patient selection for MCSD and potential future evaluation methods has been recently published by the authors' group [122]. Currently, overall outcomes after MCSD implantation are severely limited. Therefore the benefit of this therapeutic modality will likely benefit only those patients whose likelihood of survival at 1 year is less than 50%. Patients requiring inotropic support in the REMATCH study population at the time of MCSD implantation showed the highest likelihood of benefit in terms of survival and improved quality of life, whereas patients without inotropic infusions had a tendency to higher survival rates with and without MCSD [78]. The new US

Interagency Registry for Mechanical Circulatory Support registry may continue contributing with data as the ISHLT MCSD database. To better identify the urgency of the MCSD-implant recommendation and also risk-stratify patients and estimate their survival benefit from MCSD-implantation, the classification proposed by the US Interagency Registry for Mechanical Circulatory Support proposes to aggregate patients failing medical treatment into seven distinct levels. Level 1, "crash and burn," indicates that the patient needs a definitive intervention within hours. Patients have refractory life-threatening hypotension with critical organ hypoperfusion. Level 2, "sliding on inotropes," patients are those that require a definitive intervention within days and involve patients with declining function despite intravenous support. Level 3, "dependent stability," patients require a definitive intervention electively over a period of weeks. These are patients whose clinical status is stable under inotropic support but these drugs cannot be discontinued. Level 4, "Frequent flyer," identifies a subgroup of patients that requires a definitive intervention electively over a period of months as long as treatment episodes restores stable baseline, including nutritional status. Level 5, "housebound" denotes patients that are limited to daily living activities predominantly within their house. The time of implantation in these patients is variable and depends on maintenance of nutrition, organ function, and activity level. Patients in level 6 are labeled as "walking wounded." The time expected to require MCSD implantation is also variable and depends on maintenance of nutrition, organ function, and activity level as in Level 5, but patients are comfortable with daily living activities and out-of-house general activities. Patients in level 7 are stable under medical therapy with only mild limitation of clinical activities, and therefore transplantation or circulatory support may not be indicated. The modifier factors "arrhythmia" (refractory/repetitive ventricular tachycardia or fibrillation) and "angina" can denote additional stages for each condition [123]. An evaluation/reassessment approach by a multidisciplinary group is presented in Fig. 3. A stepped selection algorithm [124,125] starts with the encounter between the patient and the team which during the evaluation process will assess important issues including the evaluation of a possible end-of-life situation; the possibility to recompensate the patient; the possibility of benefit from

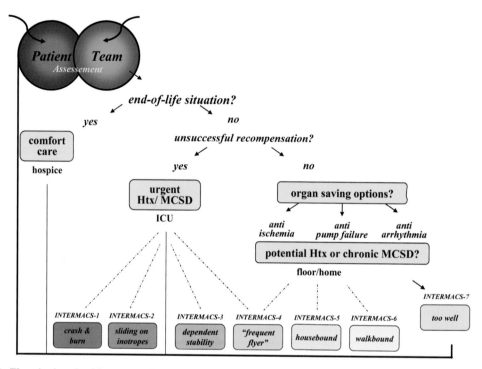

Fig. 3. The selection algorithm starts with the encounter between patient and team, and is followed by a stepwise evaluation of important issues including: (1) is an end-of-life situation present? (2) Can the patient be recompensated? (3) After neurohormonal blockade initiation, are there organ-saving options including revascularization, contractility enhancement, and antiarrhythmia therapy? (4) Is the patient a suitable candidate for heart replacement options including mechanical circulatory support and heart transplantation? (*From* Deng MC, Naka Y. Mechanical circulatory support therapy in advanced heart failure. London: Imperial College Press; 2007. p. 30; with permission.)

organ-saving strategies including revascularization, contractility enhancement, and antiarrhythmic therapy; and the suitability for heart replacement options including mechanical circulatory support and heart transplantation. Although a likelihood of recovery is foreseen, alert should rise to thoroughly and continuously reassess the possibility for MCSD explantation before proceeding to orthotopic heart transplantation. Serial echocardiographic evaluation during full support or partial unload, exercise testing, and clinical variables can be helpful in assessing this possibility. Most likely patients who have short-term history of end-stage heart failure will have the higher likelihood to recover (ie, acute myocarditis, peripartum cardiomyopahty). Genomic markers of recovery are being studied, and pharmacologic strategies have been suggested of potential benefit [126].

Improvement of accessibility to assist devices therapy

Therapy with mechanical assist devices as bridge to transplantation may spare suitable recipients and therefore make heart transplantation available for patients that otherwise seem to be to too sick to undergo transplantation. The cost of long-term left ventricular assist device implantation is commensurate with other life-saving organ transplantation procedures like liver transplantation. As an evolving technology, there are several opportunities for improvement that will likely reduce costs in the future. In the REMATCH study, the mean cost for the initial implant-related hospitalization was $210,187 ± $193,295. When implantation hospitalization costs were compared between hospital survivors and nonsurvivors, the mean costs increased from $159,271 ± $106,423 to $315,015 ± $278,713, and the average annual readmission cost per patient for the overall cohort was $105,326. A recent cost analysis of the use of left ventricular assist devices as an alternative to transplantation in the post-REMATCH era was completed in 23 consecutive patients that received a HeartMate XVE pump implanted. They evaluated survival to discharge during the implantation hospitalization, hospital length of stay and hospital costs, and compared them with outcomes reported from the RE-MATCH trial. Mean hospital costs for post-REMATCH patients were significantly lower in comparison to REMATCH patients when measured from implantation to discharge. This data showed a 40% reduction in cost from $210,187 to $128,084. Outcomes with use of left ventricular assist device as destination therapy have improved in the post-REMATCH era, including significantly lower hospital costs as well as strong trends toward better survival to hospital discharge and shorter average length of stay. Currently long-term results of MCSD makes this therapy a definite valid option only for patients who are not suitable candidates for heart transplantation [127].

Improvement of heart transplantation outcomes

Improving heart transplant management

The ISHLT database [3] has shown that over the last decade improvements has been achieved to reduce mortality mainly due to improve of the early posttransplant management during the first year after transplantation. Mortality rate of 77% at first year posttransplantation for the 1982 to 1988 period, improved to 85% in the 1999 to 2004 period. Thereafter, the slope of the curve remains far from reaching that of the normal population with an average life expectancy of 10.2 years. Chronic cardiac allograft rejection/vasculopathy still remains as the Achilles-heal of long-term management with 30% to 50% incidence at 5 years [3,128]; and Neoplasias, most commonly of the skin tissue are also a major cause of long-term mortality possible related to immunossupression levels. Possibilities to refine the management of heart transplantation is a new open window after having entered the genomic era. A novel approach to the clinical management of heart transplantation was introduced early this year by the Cardiac Allograft Rejection Gene expression Observational (CARGO) study group. The CARGO study investigated gene expression profiles of peripheral blood mononuclear

cells in cardiac transplant recipients to discriminate ISHLT grade 0/0R rejection (quiescence) from moderate/severe rejection (ISHLT > 3A/2R). Posttransplant patients at eight centers were followed prospectively with blood sampling and endomyocardial biopsies. Known alloimmune pathways and leukocyte microarrays identified candidate genes that derived in a 20-gene test sensible to distinguish rejection from quiescence [124,125]. Endomyocardial biopsy has been for the last two decades the gold standard method to guide therapy after heart transplantation. The evaluation of a subset of 827 biopsies from 273 patients identified from eight centers participating in the Cardiac Allograft Gene Expression Observational Study. Each case was reviewed in a blinded manner by three study pathologists in the absence of clinical data. Study pathologists were significantly more likely than local pathologists to diagnose ISHLT Grade 0, 1A, and 3B rejection and significantly less likely to diagnose ISHLT Grade 1B, 2, and 3A rejection. Concordance between local and study pathologists was lowest for grade 2 (17% agreement). [129] This report exemplifies an imperfect control used as a gold standard to base patient monitoring. Currently two ongoing studies, the CARGO II aimed to continue developing gene expression based monitoring of the cardiac allograft with molecular classifiers and the Invasive Monitoring Attenuation through gene Expression (IMAGE) study which will include over 500 patients to answer the question whether a validated gene test (Allo-Mapmolecular testing, XDx. Inc., Brisbane, California) compares to a nonvalidated endomyocardial biopsy based monitoring, in a noninferiority study design [130]. The first clinical experience of molecular monitoring for heart transplant patients reflected the findings of the original CARGO study, which has been recently published [131,132].

Improving selection criteria for patients that will likely benefit from specific allocation strategies based on current evidence

In the United States, currently approximately 75% of heart transplantations are performed in UNOS status 1 patients, whereas only 25% are performed in UNOS status 2 patients. Current evidence arises from the comparisons of waiting list outcomes and the reported registries and intervention clinical trials. Figs. 1 and 2 depict the effect of medical treatment (as defined by major clinical trials), patients in the UNOS/OPTN waiting list (stratified as status 1A, 1B, and 2) and heart transplantation. Based on these observations, heart transplantation might not likely provide benefits to patients listed under UNOS status 1B or 2 criteria. Patients that can be compensated with beta-blockers, resynchronization/defibrillator therapy (ie, COPERNICUS, COMPANION type of patients), will probably not retain benefit from transplantation. Patients included in the UNOS 1B category may remain stable and retain benefit from accurately implemented medical treatment or worsen and be refractory to medical treatment. Patients with the most advanced forms of end-stage heart failure (ie, ESSENTIAL, REMATCH) seems to have a greater risk of mortality in comparison to patients receiving a transplant and therefore, likely to get benefit. Therefore, transplantation benefit may need to be compared against the likelihood of benefit after recompensation and implementation of optimal medical treatment. The benefit of heart transplantation was suggested requiring to be tested in a randomized clinical trial, although ethical arguments would make this possibility unlikely to happen [133].

Improving heart transplant donation and allocation policy

In the United States, allocation systems moved toward a system that favors medical urgency over waiting time [134–136], and the policy on organ donation is based both on previous consent of the potential donor and on the consent of the donor's family. The allocation system seems to be responsive to the observations of outcomes based on the UNOS data and probably risk assessment may yet be improved. Different to the United States, other countries of which Spain got the leading role and highest rate of availability of organ donors, organ donation policies relies on the principle of presumed consent (ie, people who have not expressly opposed donating their organs are presumed eligible for donation). This fact, the strong infrastructure for organ procurement and plan of public education, is what has enhanced their donor rates. In 1999, Spain had an organ-donation rate of 33.6 organ donors per million people while in the same year, the United States had 21.8 per million [137,138]. Donation and allocation policies should be continuously monitored to offer the largest number of donors for the largest number of patients that might get benefit from this therapeutic modality. It was suggested that the high Spanish organ donation rates are largely

attributable to increased use of older donors and that in fact, using similar proportions of older donors in the United States would increase the donor pool by almost 40% [137]. In fact, in the United States, increasingly more hospitals are gaining flexibility to extend the selection of patients and donor organs with extended criteria. Alternate waiting list strategies have been evaluated in selected patients who did not meet criteria for standard listing for heart transplantation. Listing more critically ill patients and the use of so-called "marginal donor hearts," driven by increasing cardiac donor scarcity, is associated with higher postoperative risk. The outcomes of cardiac transplantation using older donors was retrospectively reviewed at Columbia University on 479 adult heart transplant recipients, 352 status I patients, and 534 status II patients enrolled on a waiting list between 1992 and 1999. Of all donors, 20% were 40 to 50 years old and 8% were 50 years or older. The risk of 6-month mortality on the waiting list for patients who were not transplanted significantly outweighed the risk of transplanting patients with a heart from donors over 40 years old. Recipients of cardiac allografts from donors younger than 40 years old had a 1-month mortality rate of 5%, in contrast to 13% and 22% in those receiving allografts from donors 40 to 50 years old and 50 years old and greater, respectively. Donor age did not influence long-term survival or frequency of rejections; however, it did correlate with the early presence of transplant-related coronary artery disease [139]. In a single center study, 37 patients (14.3%) meeting alternate list criteria including age greater than 65 years, amyloidosis, severe diabetes mellitus and peripheral vascular disease, human immunodeficiency virus or high-risk retransplant were included. The average age of alternate list donors was 41.2 ± 13.9 years. There was no posttransplant survival advantage for standard list recipient. Currently, there are no data comparing mechanical assist device in patients out bounding the age limits currently established for heart transplantation listing; although there is consensus for these patients to be eligible for MCSD destination therapy.

Summary

Based on data currently available, heart transplantation most likely will continue as the therapy of choice for heart transplant recipients who have advanced heart failure refractory to medical treatment in the absence of contraindications (ie, UNOS status 1A). Evolving approaches in all fields of transplantation does not allow making the distinction of a role of transplantation against new therapeutic modalities that might become readily available as the costs gets lower and therefore available to the whole diverse heart-failure population. Currently MCSD implantation is limited to populations that have high gross income and well-supported health systems and is still far behind heart transplantation to be readily available for weaker economies or to provide comparable benefit to patients currently considered eligible for heart transplantation or medical treatment. At the same time, we are currently in the era of evidence-based medicine. No randomized data compared heart transplantation to identify specific groups of patients that will have the greatest benefit from one or other treatment and the extension of listing criteria with patients increasingly being selected under severer conditions. The ISHLT/ UNOS database can be queried for outcomes, but it holds the known limitations that applies for registries, which has not been designed to assess the effect of cardiac transplantation on survival of patients who have heart failure. The development and implementation of new medical knowledge will require decades and therefore continuous efforts by the coming generations to develop research in all these areas within the new directions of medical knowledge leading to improvement of clinical outcomes and a personalized medical management. The development of a predictive, preemptive, personalized and participatory medicine reflected by the NIH initiative in the new genomic era characterized by high-throughput information systems will probably lead to important changes and, years from now, we will keep formulating the question, *"Heart Transplantation, any role left?"*

References

[1] Hunt SA, Rider AK, Stinson EB, et al. Does cardiac transplantation prolong life and improve its quality? An updated report. Circulation 1976;54(6 Suppl):III56–60.

[2] Mudge GH, Goldstein S, Addonizio LJ, et al. 24th Bethesda conference: cardiac transplantation. Task force 3: recipient guidelines/prioritization. J Am Coll Cardiol 1993;22(1):21–3.

[3] Taylor DO, Edwards LB, Boucek MM, et al. International Society for Heart and Lung Transplantation. Registry of the International Society for Heart and Lung Transplantation: twenty-third official adult heart transplantation report–2006. J Heart Lung Transplant 2006;25:869–79.

[4] Mancini DM, Eisen H, Kussmaul W, et al. Value of peak exercise oxygen consumption for optimal timing of cardiac transplantation in ambulatory patients with heart failure. Circulation 1991;83:778–86.

[5] Aaronson KD, Schwartz JS, Chen TM, et al. Development and prospective validation of a clinical index to predict survival in ambulatory patients referred for cardiac transplant evaluation. Circulation 1997;95:2660–7.

[6] Deng MC, De Meester JM, Smits JM, et al. Effect of receiving a heart transplant: analysis of a national cohort entered on to a waiting list, stratified by heart failure severity. Comparative outcome and clinical profiles in transplantation (COCPIT) study group. BMJ 2000;321:540–5.

[7] Deng MC, Edwards LB, Hertz MI, et al. International Society for Heart and Lung Transplantation. Mechanical circulatory support device database of the International Society for Heart and Lung Transplantation: third annual report–2005. J Heart Lung Transplant 2005;24:1182–7.

[8] Butler J, Khadim G, Paul KM, et al. Selection of patients for heart transplantation in the current era of heart failure therapy. J Am Coll Cardiol 2004;43(5):787–93.

[9] Freudenberger RS, Kim J, Tawfik I, et al. Optimal medical therapy is superior to transplantation for the treatment of class I, II, and III heart failure: a decision analytic approach. Circulation 2006; 114(1 Suppl):I62–6.

[10] Jimenez J, Bennett Edwards L, Higgins R, et al. Should stable UNOS status 2 patients be transplanted? J Heart Lung Transplant 2005;24:178–83.

[11] Rose EA, Gelijns AC, Moskowitz AJ, et al. Randomized evaluation of mechanical assistance for the treatment of congestive heart failure (REMATCH) Study Group. Long-term mechanical left ventricular assistance for end-stage heart failure. N Engl J Med 2001;345:1435–43.

[12] Swedberg K, Kjekshus J. Effects of enalapril on mortality in severe congestive heart failure: results of the Cooperative North Scandinavian enalapril survival study (CONSENSUS). N Engl J Med 1987;316:1429–35.

[13] Swedberg K, Kjekshus J, Snapinn S. Long-term survival in severe heart failure in patients treated with enalapril. Ten year follow-up of CONSENSUS I. Eur Heart J 1999;20(2):136–9.

[14] Cohn JN, Johnson G, Ziesche S, et al. A comparison of enalapril with hydralazine-isosorbide dinitrate in the treatment of chronic congestive heart failure. N Engl J Med 1991;325(5):303–10.

[15] SOLVD investigators. Effect of enalapril on survival in patients with reduced left ventricular ejection fractions and congestive heart failure. The SOLVD investigators. N Engl J Med 1991;325(5): 293–302.

[16] AIRE investigators. Effect of ramipril on mortality and morbidity of survivors of acute myocardial infarction with clinical evidence of heart failure. The Acute Infarction Ramipril Efficacy (AIRE) study investigators. Lancet 1993;342(8875):821–8.

[17] Waagstein F, Hjalmarson A, Varnauskas E, et al. Effect of chronic beta-adrenergic receptor blockade in congestive cardiomyopathy. Br Heart J 1975; 37(10):1022–36.

[18] Packer M, Bristow MR, Cohn JN, et al. The effect of carvedilol on morbidity and mortality in patients with chronic heart failure. U.S. Carvedilol Heart Failure Study Group. N Engl J Med 1996; 334(21):1349–55.

[19] CIBIS-II investigators. The Cardiac Insufficiency Bisoprolol Study II (CIBIS-II): a randomized trial. Lancet 1999;353(9146):9–13.

[20] MERIT investigators. Effect of metoprolol CR/XL in chronic heart failure: Metoprolol CR/XL Randomised Intervention Trial in Congestive Heart Failure (MERIT-HF). Lancet 1999;353(9169):2001–7.

[21] Packer M, Coats AJ, Fowler MB, et al. Carvedilol Prospective Randomized Cumulative Survival Study Group. Effect of carvedilol on survival in severe chronic heart failure. N Engl J Med 2001; 344(22):1651–8.

[22] Poole-Wilson PA, Swedberg K, Cleland JG, et al. Carvedilol or Metoprolol European Trial Investigators. Comparison of carvedilol and metoprolol on clinical outcomes in patients with chronic heart failure in the Carvedilol or Metoprolol European Trial (COMET): randomized controlled trial. Lancet 2003;362(9377):7–13.

[23] Pitt B, Zannad F, Remme WJ, et al. The effect of spironolactone on morbidity and mortality in patients with severe heart failure. Randomized aldactone evaluation study investigators. N Engl J Med 1999;341:709–17.

[24] Pitt B, Remme W, Zannad F, et al. Eplerenone post-acute myocardial infarction heart failure efficacy and survival study investigators. Eplerenone, a selective aldosterone blocker, in patients with left ventricular dysfunction after myocardial infarction. N Engl J Med 2003;348(14):1309–21.

[25] Pitt B, Gheorghiade M, Zannad F, et al. On behalf of the EPHESUS Investigators. Evaluation of eplerenone in the subgroup of EPHESUS patients with baseline left ventricular ejection fraction <or=30%. Eur J Heart Fail 2006;8(3):295–301.

[26] Cohn JN, Tognoni G, for the Valsartan Heart Failure Trial Investigators A randomized trial of the angiotensin- receptor blocker valsartan in chronic heart failure. N Engl J Med 2001;345: 1667–75.

[27] Granger CB, McMurray JJ, Yusuf S, et al. CHARM Investigators and Committees. Effects of candesartan in patients with chronic heart failure and reduced left-ventricular systolic function intolerant to angiotensin-converting-enzyme inhibitors: the CHARM-alternative trial. Lancet 2003; 362(9386):772–6.

[28] McMurray JJ, Ostergren J, Swedberg K, et al. CHARM Investigators and Committees. Effects of candesartan in patients with chronic heart failure and reduced left-ventricular systolic function taking angiotensin-converting-enzyme inhibitors: the CHARM-added trial. Lancet 2003;362(9386): 767–71.

[29] Cohn JN, Goldstein SO, Greenberg BH, et al. A dose-dependent increase in mortality with vesnarinone among patients with severe heart failure. Vesnarinone trial investigators. N Engl J Med 1998; 339:1810–6.

[30] Feldman AM, Bristow MR, Parmley WW, et al. Effects of vesnarinone on morbidity and mortality in patients with heart failure. Vesnarinone study group. N Engl J Med 1993;329:149–55.

[31] Ryden L, for the Xamoterol in Severe Heart Failure Study Group. Xamoterol in severe heart failure. The Xamoterol in severe heart failure study group. Lancet 1990;336:1–6.

[32] Hampton JR, van Veldhuisen DJ, Kleber FX, et al. Randomised study of effect of ibopamine on survival in patients with advanced severe heart failure. Second Prospective Randomised Study of Ibopamine on Mortality and Efficacy (PRIME II) investigators. Lancet 1997;349:971–7.

[33] Packer M, Carver JR, Rodeheffer RJ, et al. Effect of oral milrinone on mortality in severe chronic heart failure. The PROMISE study research group. N Engl J Med 1991;325:1468–75.

[34] Packer M, Caspi A, Charlon V, et al. Multicenter, double-blind, placebo-controlled study of long-term endothelin blockade with bosentan in chronic heart failure: results of the REACH-1 trial. Circulation 1998;98(Suppl I):I–3. [abstract].

[35] Califf RM, Adams KF, McKenna WJ, et al. A randomized controlled trial of epoprostenol therapy for severe congestive heart failure: The Flolan International Randomized Survival Trial (FIRST). Am Heart J 1997;134:44–54.

[36] Brozena SC, Twomey C, Goldberg LR, et al. A prospective study of continuous intravenous milrinone therapy for status IB patients awaiting heart transplant at home. J Heart Lung Transplant 2004;23(9):1082–6.

[37] Upadya S, Lee FA, Saldarriaga C, et al. Home continuous positive inotropic infusion as a bridge to cardiac transplantation in patients with end-stage heart failure. J Heart Lung Transplant 2004;23(4): 466–72.

[38] Lowes BD, Higginbotham M, Petrovich L, et al. Low-dose enoximone improves exercise capacity in chronic heart failure. Enoximone study group. J Am Coll Cardiol 2000;36(2):501–8.

[39] Metra M. European Society of Cardiology Congress 2005. Stockholm (Sweden). September 4–7, 2005.

[40] Hunt SA. American college of cardiology; American heart association task force on practice guidelines (writing committee to update the 2001 guidelines for the evaluation and management of heart failure). ACC/AHA 2005 guideline update for the diagnosis and management of chronic heart failure in the adult: a report of the American College of Cardiology/American Heart Association Task Force on Practice Guidelines (Writing Committee to Update the 2001 Guidelines for the Evaluation and Management of Heart Failure). J Am Coll Cardiol 2005;46(6): e1–82.

[41] Gheorghiade M, De Luca L, Bonow RO. Neurohormonal inhibition in heart failure: insights from recent clinical trials. Am J Cardiol 2005;96(12A): 3L–9L.

[42] Cazeau S, Leclercq C, Lavergne T, et al. Multisite Stimulation in Cardiomyopathies (MUSTIC) study investigators. Effects of multisite biventricular pacing in patients with heart failure and intraventricular conduction delay. N Engl J Med 2001; 344:873–80.

[43] Abraham WT, Fisher WG, Smith AL, et al. MIRACLE Study Group. Multicenter cardiac resynchronization in chronic heart failure. N Engl J Med 2002;346(24):1845–53.

[44] Bristow MR, Saxon LA, Boehmer J, et al. Comparison of medical therapy, pacing, and defibrillation in heart failure (COMPANION) investigators. Cardiac-resynchronization therapy with or without an implantable defibrillator in advanced chronic heart failure. N Engl J Med 2004;350(21):2140–50.

[45] Cleland JG, Coletta AP, Lammiman M, et al. Clinical trials update from the European Society of Cardiology meeting 2005: CARE-HF extension study, ESSENTIAL, CIBIS-III, S-ICD, ISSUE-2, STRIDE-2, SOFA, IMAGINE, PREAMI, SIRIUS-II and ACTIVE. Eur J Heart Fail 2005;7(6):1070–5.

[46] Cleland JG, Daubert JC, Erdmann E, et al. Cardiac Resynchronization-Heart Failure (CARE-HF) study investigators. The effect of cardiac resynchronization on morbidity and mortality in heart failure. N Engl J Med 2005;352(15):1539–49.

[47] Bardy GH, Lee KL, Mark DB, et al. Sudden cardiac death in heart failure trial (SCD-HeFT) investigators. Amiodarone or an implantable cardioverter-defibrillator for congestive heart failure. N Engl J Med 2005;352:225–37.

[48] Moss AJ, Hall WJ, Cannom DS, et al. Improved survival with an implanted defibrillator in patients with coronary disease at high risk for ventricular arrhythmia. Multicenter Automatic Defibrillator Implantation Trial Investigators. N Engl J Med 1996;335:1933–40.

[49] Moss AJ, Zareba W, Hall WJ, et al. Multicenter Automatic Defibrillator Implantation Trial II Investigators. Prophylactic implantation of a defibrillator in patients with myocardial infarction and reduced ejection fraction. N Engl J Med 2002;346: 877–83.

[50] BARI investigators. Comparison of coronary bypass surgery with angioplasty in patients with multivessel disease. The bypass angioplasty revascularization investigation (BARI) investigators. N Engl J Med 1996;335:217–25.

[51] Morrison DA, Sethi G, Sacks J, et al. Angina with extremely serious operative mortality evaluation (AWESOME). Percutaneous coronary intervention versus coronary artery bypass graft surgery for patients with medically refractory myocardial ischemia and risk factors for adverse outcomes with bypass: a multicenter, randomized trial. Investigators of the Department of Veterans Affairs Cooperative Study #385, the Angina With Extremely Serious Operative Mortality Evaluation (AWESOME). J Am Coll Cardiol 2001;38(1):143–9.

[52] Hannan EL, Racz MJ, Walford G, et al. Long-term outcomes of coronary-artery bypass grafting versus stent implantation. N Engl J Med 2005;352: 2174–83.

[53] Smith SC Jr, Feldman TE, Hirshfeld JW Jr, et al. American College of Cardiology/American Heart Association Task Force on Practice Guidelines; ACC/AHA/SCAI Writing Committee to Update 2001 Guidelines for Percutaneous Coronary Intervention. ACC/AHA/SCAI 2005 guideline update for percutaneous coronary intervention: a report of the American College of Cardiology/American Heart Association Task Force on Practice Guidelines (ACC/AHA/SCAI Writing Committee to Update 2001 Guidelines for Percutaneous Coronary Intervention). Circulation 2006;113:e166–286.

[54] Joyce D, Loebe M, Noon GP, et al. Revascularization and ventricular restoration in patients with ischemic heart failure: the STICH trial. Curr Opin Cardiol 2003;6:454–7.

[55] STICH Trial. Available at: https://www.stichtrial.org/. Accessed November, 2006.

[56] Veenhuyzen GD, Singh SN, McAreavey D, et al. Prior coronary artery bypass surgery and risk of death among patients with ischemic left ventricular dysfunction. Circulation 2001;104:1489–93.

[57] Kron IL, Flanagan TL, Blackbourne LH, et al. Coronary revascularization rather than cardiac transplantation for chronic ischemic cardiomyopathy. Ann Surg 1989;210:348–54.

[58] Winkel E, Piccione W. Coronary artery bypass surgery in patients with left ventricular dysfunction: Candidate selection and perioperative care. J Heart Lung Transplant 1997;16:S19–24.

[59] Di Carli MF, Asgarzadie F, Schelbert HR, et al. Quantitative relation between myocardial viability and improvement in heart failure symptoms after revascularization in patients with ischemic cardiomyopathy. Circulation 1995;92:3436–44.

[60] Elefteriades JA, Tolis G, Levi E, et al. Coronary artery bypass grafting in severe left ventricular

dysfunction: excellent survival and improved EF and functional state. J Am Coll Cardiol 1993;22: 1411–7.

[61] Hausmann H, Topp H, Siniawski H, et al. Decision-making in end-stage coronary artery disease: revascularization or heart transplantation? Ann Thorac Surg 1997;64:1296–302.

[62] Mickleborough LL, Maruyama H, Takagi Y, et al. Results of revascularization in patients with severe left ventricular dysfunction. Circulation 1995; 92(Suppl II):S73–9.

[63] Olson PS, Kassis E, Niebuhr-Jorgensen U. Coronary artery bypass surgery in patients with severe left ventricular dysfunction. Thorac Cardiovasc Surg 1993;41:118–20.

[64] Oz MC, Gelijns AC, Miller L, et al. Left ventricular assist devices as permanent heart failure therapy: the price of progress. Ann Surg 2003;238(4):577–83.

[65] Dreyfus G, Duboc D, Blasco A, et al. Coronary surgery can be an alternative to heart transplantation in selected patients with end-stage ischemic heart disease. Eur J Cardiothorac Surg 1993;7: 482–8.

[66] Lansman SL, Cohen M, Galla JD, et al. Coronary bypass with ejection fraction of 0.20 or less using centigrade cardioplegia: longterm follow-up. Ann Thorac Surg 1993;56:480–6.

[67] Tjan TDT, Kondruweit M, Scheld HH, et al. The bad ventricle—revascularization versus transplantation. Thorac Cardiovasc Surg 2000;48:1–6.

[68] Bolling SF, Pagani FD, Deeb GM, et al. Intermediate-term outcome of mitral reconstruction in cardiomyopathy. Thorac Cardiovasc Surg 1998;115: 381–6.

[69] Wu AH, Aaronson KD, Bolling SF, et al. Impact of mitral valve annuloplasty on mortality risk in patients with mitral regurgitation and left ventricular systolic dysfunction. J Am Coll Cardiol 2005;45: 381–7.

[70] Acker MA, Bolling S, Shemin R, et al. Acorn mitral valve surgery in heart failure: insights from the acorn clinical trial. J Thorac Cardiovasc Surg 2006;132:568–77.

[71] Bonow RO, Carabellow BA, Chatterjee K, et al. ACC/AHA 2006 Practice guidelines for the management of patients with valvular heart disease: executive summary: a report of the American College of cardiology/american heart association task force on practice guidelines (writing committee to revise the 1998 guidelines for the management of patients with valvular heart disease) developed in collaboration with the society of cardiovascular anesthesiologists endorsed by the society for cardiovascular angiography and interventions and the society of thoracic surgeons. J Am Coll Cardiol 2006;4: 598–675.

[72] Connolly HM, Oh JK, Schaff HV, et al. Severe aortic stenosis with low transvalvular gradient and severe left ventricular dysfunction: result of aortic valve replacement in 52 patients. Circulation 2000;101:1940–6.

[73] Pereira JJ, Lauer MS, Bashir M, et al. Survival after aortic valve replacement for severe aortic stenosis with low transvalvular gradients and severe left ventricular dysfunction. J Am Coll Cardiol 2002; 39(8):1356–63.

[74] Chukwuemeka A, Rao V, Armstrong S, et al. Aortic valve replacement: a safe and durable option in patients with impaired left ventricular systolic function. Eur J Cardiothorac Surg 2006;29:133–8.

[75] Athanasuleas CL, Stanley AW Jr, Buckberg GD, et al. Surgical anterior ventricular endocardial restoration (SAVER) in the dilated remodeled ventricle after anterior myocardial infarction. J Am Coll Cardiol 2001;37:1199–209.

[76] Athanasuleas CL, Buckberg GD, Stanley AW, et al. RESTORE group. Surgical ventricular restoration in the treatment of congestive heart failure due to post-infarction ventricular dilation. J Am Coll Cardiol 2004;44:1439–45.

[77] Stevenson LW. Left ventricular assist devices as destination therapy for end-stage heart failure. Curr Treat Options Cardiovasc Med 2004;6:471–9.

[78] Young JB, Rogers JG, Portner PM, et al. Bridge to eligibility: LVAS-support in patients with relative contraindications to transplantation. J Heart Lung Transplant 2005;24:S75.

[79] Jurmann MJ, Weng Y, Drews T, et al. Permanent mechanical circulatory support in patients of advanced age. Eur J Cardiothorac Surg 2004;25: 610–8.

[80] Siegenthaler MP, Westaby S, Frazier OH, et al. Advanced heart failure: study feasibility of long term continuous axial flow pump support. Eur Heart J 2005;26:1031–8.

[81] Holman WL, Park SJ, Long JW, et al. Infection in permanent circulatory support: experience from the REMATCH trial. J Heart Lung Transplant 2004;23:1359–65.

[82] Hood L, Heath JR, Phelps ME, et al. Systems biology and new technologies enable predictive and preventative medicine. Science 2004;306:640–3.

[83] Simon D, Fischer S, Grossman A, et al. Left ventricular assist device-related infection: treatment and outcome. Clin Infect Dis 2005;40:1108–15.

[84] Lazar RM, Shapiro PA, Jaski BE, et al. Neurological events during long-term mechanical circulatory support for heart failure: the Randomized Evaluation of Mechanical Assistance for the Treatment of Congestive Heart Failure (REMATCH) experience. Circulation 2004;109:2423–7.

[85] Martin J, Siegenthaler MP, Friesewinkel O, et al. Implantable left ventricular assist device for treatment of pulmonary hypertension in candidates for orthotopic heart transplantation: a preliminary study. Eur J Cardiothorac Surg 2004;25:971–7.

[86] Salzberg SP, Lachat ML, von Harbou K, et al. Normalization of high pulmonary vascular resistance

with LVAD support in heart transplantation candidates. Eur J Cardiothorac Surg 2005;27: 222–5.

[87] Dowling RD, Park SJ, Pagani FD, et al. Heart-Mate VE LVAS design enhancements and its impact on device reliability. Eur J Cardiothorac Surg 2004;25:958–63.

[88] Birks EJ, Tansley PD, Yacoub MH, et al. Incidence and clinical management of life-threatening left ventricular assist device failure. J Heart Lung Transplant 2004;23:964–9.

[89] Mehra MR, Kobashigawa J, Starling R, et al. Listing criteria for heart transplantation: International Society for Heart and Lung Transplantation guidelines for the care of cardiac transplant candidates—2006. J Heart Lung Transplant 2006;25(9):1024–42.

[90] Deng MC, Smits JM, Packer M. Selecting patients for heart transplantation: which patients are too well for transplant? Curr Opin Cardiol 2002; 17(2):137–44.

[91] Zugck C, Haunstetter A, Kruger C, et al. Impact of beta-blocker treatment on the prognostic value of currently used risk predictors in congestive heart failure. J Am Coll Cardiol 2002;39(10):1615–22.

[92] Lund LH, Aaronson KD, Mancini DM. Predicting survival in ambulatory patients with severe heart failure on beta-blocker therapy. Am J Cardiol 2003;92(11):1350–4.

[93] O'Neill JO, Young JB, Pothier CE, et al. Peak oxygen consumption as a predictor of death in patients with heart failure receiving beta-blockers. Circulation 2005;111(18):2313–8.

[94] McAlister FA, Stewart S, Ferrua S, et al. Multidisciplinary strategies for the management of heart failure patients at high risk for admission: a systematic review of randomized trials. J Am Coll Cardiol 2004;44(4):810–9.

[95] Koelling TM, Johnson ML, Cody RJ, et al. Discharge education improves clinical outcomes in patients with chronic heart failure. Circulation 2005;111:179–85.

[96] Inglis SC, Pearson S, Treen S, et al. Extending the horizon in chronic heart failure. Effects of multidisciplinary, home-based intervention relative to usual care. Circulation 2006;114(23):2466–73.

[97] International HapMap Consortium. A haplotype map of the human genome. Nature 2005;437: 1299–320.

[98] Packer M, Abraham WT, Mehra MR, et al. Prospective Evaluation and Identification of Cardiac Decompensation by ICG Test (PREDICT) study investigators and coordinators. Utility of impedance cardiography for the identification of short-term risk of clinical decompensation in stable patients with chronic heart failure. J Am Coll Cardiol 2006;47(11):2245–52.

[99] Bourge RC. Case Studies in advanced monitoring with the Chronicle device. Rev Cardiovasc Med 2006;7(Suppl 1):S56–61.

[100] Packer M, Califf RM, Konstam MA, et al. Comparison of omapatrilat and enalapril in patients with chronic heart failure: the Omapatrilat Versus Enalapril Randomized Trial of Utility in Reducing Events (OVERTURE). Circulation 2002;106(8):920–6.

[101] Swedberg K, Bristow MR, Cohn JN, et al. Moxonidine Safety and Efficacy (MOXSE) Investigators. Effects of sustained-release moxonidine, an imidazoline agonist, on plasma norepinephrine in patients with chronic heart failure. Circulation 2002; 105(15):1797–803.

[102] Bozkurt B, Torre-Amione G, Warren MS, et al. Results of targeted anti-tumor necrosis factor therapy with etanercept (ENBREL) in patients with advanced heart failure. Circulation 2001;103(8): 1044–7.

[103] Rich S, McLaughlin VV. Endothelian receptor blockers in cardiovascular disease. Circulation 2003;108(18):2184–90.

[104] O'Connor CM, Gattis WA, Adams KF Jr, et al. Randomized Intravenous TeZosentan Study-4 Investigators. Tezosentan in patients with acute heart failure and acute coronary syndromes: results of the Randomized Intravenous TeZosentan Study-4 (RITZ-4). J Am Coll Cardiol 2003;41(9):1452–7.

[105] Kaluski E, Kobrin I, Zimlickman R, et al. RITZ-5: randomized intravenous TeZosentan (an endothelin-A/B antagonist) for the treatment of pulmonary edema: a prospective, multicenter, double-blind, placebo-controlled study. J Am Coll Cardiol 2003;41(2):204–10.

[106] Teerlink JR, McMurray JJ, Bourge RC, et alVERITAS Investigators. Tezosentan in patients with acute heart failure: design of the Value on Endothelin Receptor Inhibitor with Tezosentan in Acute Heart Failure Study (VERITAS). Am Heart J 2005;150(1):46–53.

[107] Anand I, McMurray JJ, Cohn JN, et alEARTH Investigators. Long-terms effects of darusentan on left ventricular remodeling and clinical outcomes in the EndothelinA Receptor Antagonist Trial in Heart Failure (EARTH): randomized, double-blind, placebo-controlled trial. Lancet 2004; 364(9431):347–54.

[108] Lauscher TF, Enseleit F, Pacher R, et al. Hemodynamic and neurohumoral effects of selective endothelin A (ET(A)) receptor blockade in chronic heart failure: the Heart Failure ET(A) Receptor Blockade Trial (HEAT). Circulation 2002; 106(21):2666–72.

[109] Deswal A, Bozkurt B, Seta Y, et al. Safety and efficacy of a soluble P75 tumor necrosis factor receptor (Enbrel, etanercept) in patients with advanced heart failure. Circulation 1999;99(25):3224–6.

[110] Mann DL, McMurray JJ, Packer M, et al. Targeted anticytokine therapy in patients with chronic heart failure: results of the Randomized Etanercept Worldwide Evaluation (RENEWAL). Circulation 2004;109(13):1594–602.

[111] Chung ES, Packer M, Lo KH, et al. Anti-TNF Therapy Against Congestive Heart Failure Investigators. Randomized, double-blind, placebo-controlled, pilot trial of infliximab, a chimeric monoclonal antibody to tumor necrosis factor-alpha, in patients with moderate-to-severe heart failure: results of the anti-TNF Therapy Against Congestive Heart Failure (ATTACH) trial. Circulation 2003;107(25):3133–40.

[112] Zohlnhöfer D, Ott I, Mehilli J, et al. REVIVAL-2 Investigators. Stem cell mobilization by granulocyte colony-stimulating factor in patients with acute myocardial infarction: a randomized controlled trial. JAMA 2006;295(9):1003–10.

[113] Wollert KC, Meyer GP, Lotz J, et al. Intracoronary autologous bone-marrow cell transfer after myocardial infarction: the BOOST randomised controlled clinical trial. Lancet 2004;364(9429):141–8.

[114] Strauer BE, Brehm M, Zeus T, et al. Regeneration of human infarcted heart muscle by intracoronary autologous bone marrow cell transplantation in chronic coronary artery disease: the IACT Study. J Am Coll Cardiol 2005;46(9):1651–8.

[115] Schachinger V, Erbs S, Elsasser A, et al. REPAIR-AMI Investigators. Intracoronary bone marrow-derived progenitor cells in acute myocardial infarction. N Engl J Med 2006;355(12):1210–21.

[116] Assmus B, Honold J, Schachinger V, et al. Transcoronary transplantation of progenitor cells after myocardial infarction. N Engl J Med 2006;355(12):1222–32.

[117] Lander ES, Linton LM, Birren B, et al. Initial sequencing and analysis of the human genome. Nature 2001;409:860–921.

[118] Caron PR, Mullican MD, Mashal RD, et al. Chemogenomic approaches to drug discovery. Curr Opin Chem Biol 2001;5(4):464–70.

[119] Di Bernardo D, Thompson MJ, Gardner TS, et al. Chemogenomic profiling on a genome-wide scale using reverse-engineered gene networks. Nat Biotechnol 2005;23(3):377–8.

[120] Gardner TS, di Bernardo D, Lorenz D, et al. Inferring genetic networks and identifying compound mode of action via expression profiling. Science 2003;301(5629):102–5.

[121] Cadeiras M, Von Bayern MP, Pal A, et al. Destination therapy: an alternative for end-stage heart failure patients not eligible for heart transplantation. Curr Opin Organ Transplant 2005;10:369–75.

[122] Stevenson LW. The evolving role of mechanical circulatory support in advanced heart failure. In: Frazier OH, Kirklin JK, editors. Mechanical circulatory support (ISHLT Monograph Series Volume 1). Philadelphia: Elsevier; 2006.

[123] Deng MC, Naka Y. Mechanical circulatory support therapy in advanced heart failure. World Scientific Press; 2006.

[124] Deng MC, Eisen HJ, Mehra MR, et al. Noninvasive discrimination of rejection in cardiac allograft recipients using gene expression profiling. Am J Transplant 2006;6(1):150–60.

[125] Birks EJ, Tansley PD, Hardy J, et al. Left ventricular assist device and drug therapy for the reversal of heart failure. N Engl J Med 2006;355:1873–84.

[126] Miller LW, Nelson KE, Bostic RR, et al. Hospital costs for left ventricular assist devices for destination therapy: lower costs for implantation in the post-REMATCH era. J Heart Lung Transplant 2006;25(7):778–84.

[127] Kobashigawa JA, Tobis JM, Starling RC, et al. Multicenter intravascular ultrasound validation study among heart transplant recipients: outcomes after five years. J Am Coll Cardiol 2005;45(9):1532–7.

[128] Marboe CC, Billingham M, Eisen H, et al. Nodular endocardial infiltrates (Quilty lesions) cause significant variability in diagnosis of ISHLT grade 2 and 3A rejection in cardiac allograft recipients. J Heart Lung Transplant 2005;24(7 Suppl):S219–26.

[129] Starling RC, Pham M, Valantine H, et al. Working Group on Molecular Testing in Cardiac Transplantation. Molecular testing in the management of cardiac transplant recipients: initial clinical experience. J Heart Lung Transplant 2006;25(2):1389–95.

[130] National Institutes of Health. IMAGE: a comparison of allomap molecular testing and traditional biopsy-based surveillance for heart transplant rejection. ClincalTrials.gov NCT00351559. Available at: http://clinicaltrials.gov/ct/show/NCT00351559. Accessed July 24, 2007.

[131] Stevenson LW, Miller LW, Desvigne-Nickens P, et al. Left ventricular assist device as destination for patients undergoing intravenous inotropic therapy: a subset analysis from REMATCH (Randomized Evaluation of Mechanical Assistance in Treatment of Chronic Heart Failure). Circulation 2004;110:975–81.

[132] Hunt SA. A fair way of donating hearts for transplantation. BMJ 2000;321:526–526.

[133] Gibbons RD, Meltzer D, N Duan et-al. Institute of medicine committee on organ procurement and transplantation, waiting for organ transplantation. Science 2000; 287:237–8.

[134] Goldberg LR, Jessup M. Stage B heart failure: management of asymptomatic left ventricular systolic dysfunction. Circulation 2006;113(24):2851–60.

[135] Meltzer D. Waiting for organ transplantation. Transplant Proc 2003;35(3):969–70.

[136] Chang GJ, Mahanty HD, Ascher NL, et al. Expanding the donor pool: can the Spanish model work in the United States? Am J Transplant 2003;3(10):1259–63.

[137] Gundle K. Presumed consent: an international comparison and possibilities for change in the United States. Camb Q Healthc Ethics 2005; 14(1):113–8.

[138] Lietz K, Miller LW. Left ventricular assist devices: evolving devices and indications for use in ischemic heart disease. Curr Opin Cardiol 2004; 19(6):613–8.

[139] Chen JM, Russo MJ, Hammond KM, et al. Alternate waiting list strategies for heart transplantation maximize donor organ utilization. Ann Thorac Surg 2005;80(1):224–8.

ELSEVIER
SAUNDERS

Heart Failure Clin 3 (2007) 349–367

HEART
FAILURE
CLINICS

Destination Therapy: Does Progress Depend on Left Ventricular Assist Device Development?

Manuel Prinz von Bayern, PhD, Martin Cadeiras, MD,
Mario C. Deng, MD, FACC, FESC*

College of Physicians and Surgeons, Columbia University, New York, NY, USA

Organ-saving therapies for advanced heart failure have emerged over the last two decades that have, in large randomized clinical trials, established a survival and quality of life (QoL) benefit in advanced heart failure. These include angiotensin-converting enzyme/RAAS inhibitors, beta-blockers, aldosterone blockade, defibrillators, biventricular pacers, and long-term destination mechanical circulatory support devices (MCSD). Observational data support the use of cardiac surgical interventions, including revascularization, mitral valve repair, left ventricular geometry restoration, and cardiac transplantation. The potential of gene therapy, cell transplantation, and xenotransplantation is actively being explored [1–7]. In this context, the role of MCSD therapy has evolved rapidly over the last two decades. New developments in the field achieved smaller adverse event rates but, currently, only minor improvements in survival were observed in published observational data. The authors discuss the development of MCSD as a "destination therapy" option for patients who have end-stage heart failure who were ineligible for heart transplantation as it relates to left ventricular assist device development.

Destination therapy/Randomized Evaluation of Mechanical Assistant for the Treatment of Congestive Heart Failure study results

An excellent summary of the evolution of destination MCSD therapy has recently been provided [8]. The Randomized Evaluation of Mechanical Assistance for the Treatment of Congestive Heart Failure (REMATCH) trial has established, for the first time in the mechanical circulatory support field, a survival benefit and QoL benefit from MCSD implantation in patients who have end-stage heart failure who were ineligible for cardiac transplantation, showing a 48% reduction in the risk of death from any cause in the group randomized to MCSD compared with those under optimal medical management [9]. Patients who had MCSD had a significantly greater chance of suffering serious adverse events but provided a significant improvement in QoL. The evidence of benefit has been extended in a more recent analysis of the REMATCH cohort, which supported the initial observation based on the extended follow-up beyond 2 years. In addition, a significant improvement in survival was observed for MCSD-supported patients enrolled during the second half of the trial compared with the first half, and consistently, the Minnesota Living with Heart Failure QoL score improved significantly over the course of the trial in the study group [10]. Further analysis of patients requiring inotropic support within this study population at the time of MCSD implantation showed the highest likelihood benefit for them in terms of survival and improved QoL, whereas patients not undergoing inotropic infusions had a tendency to

* Corresponding author. Division of Cardiology, Department of Medicine, Columbia University College of Physicians & Surgeons, New York Presbyterian Hospital, 622 W 168th Street PH12 Stem, Room 134, New York, NY 10032.

E-mail address: md785@columbia.edu (M.C. Deng).

1551-7136/07/$ - see front matter © 2007 Elsevier Inc. All rights reserved.
doi:10.1016/j.hfc.2007.04.007

higher survival rates with and without MCSD [11], implying that only patients who are inotrope-dependent and therefore likely have a 1-year survival probability without MCSD implantation of less than 50%; MCSD intervention will add to survival and QoL benefit [11].

Post-Randomized Evaluation of Mechanical Assistant for the Treatment of Congestive Heart Failure destination mechanical circulatory support devices regulatory and research scenario

United States regulatory scenario

After the completion of the REMATCH trial, the US Food and Drug Administration (FDA) approved the HeartMate VE (HeartMate, Thoratec, California) for destination therapy in October 2002. In October 2003, the US Centers of Medicare and Medicaid Services (CMS) approved reimbursement in a national coverage decision. Since then, more than 68 United States (US) centers have been approved for destination MCSD therapy.

The FDA monitors the total product life cycle of medical devices including early preclinical development, clinical study, marketing approval, postapproval evaluation, and development of new device generations. For the approval of newer MCSD for destination therapy after completion of the REMATCH study, the FDA is requiring a randomized comparison of MCSD against the approved (HeartMate 1) (HeartMate, Thoratec, California) assist devices [12]. In addition, the postmarket monitoring of medical devices to characterize real-world performance outside of the highly selective protocol of an investigational device exemption is required. The FDA may require such studies to be conducted as a condition of premarket approval whereby such studies can provide data that cannot be derived preapproval. Similarly, postmarket registry participation may also be requested by the CMS and can be a reimbursement criterion required by CMS in certain cases [13]. Based on a National Institutes of Health Request for Application in 2004, a mandatory MCSD-registry named INTERMACS (Interagency Registry for Mechanically Assisted Circulatory Support) was initiated for US destination implant centers. As of February 26th, 2007, INTERMACS enrolled 238 patients in 71 active centers across the US [14].

Randomized clinical trial research design

Available evidence suggest that new left ventricular assist devices promise fewer adverse events [15,16], but, currently, only minor improvements in survival have been obtained. Small treatment effects, limited patient populations, elevated cost, and the increasing number of left ventricular assist devices in development challenge the efficient conduct of premarketing clinical trials and hamper innovation [12].

The randomized evaluation of Novacor left ventricular assist system (LVAS) (World Heart Inc., Oakland, California) in a nontransplant population (RELIANT) was originally designed as a multicenter randomized clinical trial with a primary endpoint of all-cause mortality and randomized 2:1 allocation of patients into the Novacor versus HeartMate XVE (HeartMate, Thoratec, California) arm revised primary endpoint and target population due to slow recruitment. The Destination Evaluation Long-term Assist trial of the Micromed DeBakey MCSD was—also secondary to slow enrollment—suspended by the sponsor while evaluating alternatives. The destination therapy trial for the HeartMate II (HeartMate, Thoratec, California)—also designed similar to RELIANT—enrolling 200 patients, was initiated in March 2005. A multicenter destination therapy trial of the Jarvik 2000 is ongoing in Europe [17]. A single-center destination therapy trial of the VentrAssist (Ventracor Ltd., Chatswood NSW, Australia) hydrodynamically suspended centrifugal pump was initiated in Australia [18] and is now going on in North America. MCSD development and implementation delay may have roots on limited dynamics of clinical trials. It has been proposed that novel trial designs would facilitate this process. Small randomized trials would preserve the advantages of randomization and allow for a shorter enrollment period and advocate an evidence shift toward postmarketing studies [12].

The FDA regulation originated on the Medical Device Modernization Act of 1997 requires the FDA to employ the "least-burdensome" approach, one that generates the required safety and effectiveness data in the most efficient, unbiased manner. The FDA provides three paths whereby medical devices can achieve market access: demonstration of substantial equivalence to a "preamendment device" product (510[k]), premarket approval, and humanitarian device exemption. For devices that present the highest level of risk to the patient in event of failure, the stringent requirements of a premarket approval process are generally necessary. A humanitarian device exemption reduces the level of benefit that must be de-monstrated. In the European Union, except in the highest-risk device category, self-certification by the manufacturer that devices meet specified standards permits labeling with the Conformite Europenne mark to allow distribution through-out the Union; but for high-risk devices, appli-cation for labeling must first be reviewed by an independent notifying entity. Global harmoniza-tion to regulatory requirements for devices is under discussion between the FDA and foreign peer organizations as considerable advantage might accrue to the conduct of clinical trials for medical devices from a more uniform regulatory environment that crosses national borders to permit pooling of data [13].

The Interagency Registry for Mechanically Assisted Circulatory Support is an internet-based registry for all MCSD implants, supported by the National Heart, Lung, and Blood Institute [14]. The registry is a unique collaboration of academia, industry, and governmental agencies (Department of Health and Human Services Agencies, National Institutes of Health, FDA, and CMS) that may become a model for future postmarket monitoring of innovative medical devices; it will provide the robust active reporting of device performance that is often lacking with passive reporting such as the Medical Device Re-porting and MedWatch programs that the FDA currently relies on. Participation by MCSD man-ufacturers is likely to address the postmarketing requirements of FDA and fulfill CMS require-ments for reimbursement. The information generated from this registry will be valuable for defining additional applications for such devices and to direct future research [13].

Post-Randomized Evaluation of Mechanical Assistant for the Treatment of Congestive Heart Failure clinical studies

After REMATCH, other devices have also shown a benefit in the transplant ineligible pop-ulation, although they have not been tested in prospective randomized trials. A retrospective analysis in 255 Novacor assist system recipients showed similar effects as the HeartMate I device [19], whereas newer experiences with permanent axial flow MCSD demonstrated their potential to settle as a treatment option in ineligible and se-lected elderly patients who have end-stage heart failure that are ineligible for heart transplantation [16,20]. In the Third Annual ISHLT-MCSD re-port, the vast majority of patients are triaged to destination MCSD because of advanced age or se-vere comorbidities, which make them poorly suited for transplantation. Most of these patients received pulsatile MCSDs. Among the entire co-hort of destination patients, the actuarial survival was 65% at 6 months and 34% at 1 year. In the multivariable analysis for the overall group, older age remained as a major risk factor for mortality. Among patients less than 65 years of age at the time of destination therapy, the actuarial survival at 1 year was 41%; for those over the age of 65, it was less than 30% (Table 1) [21,22].

Table 1
Estimation of destination therapy mechanical circulatory support device outcomes based on pooled outcomes extracted from current publications. Clinical data and outcomes from the 2005 International Society of Heart and Lung Trans-plantation Mechanical Circulatory Support Device database report are provided for comparison

Experience	Enrollment Start date	N	Age	Male (%)	IHD (%)	EF (%)	Survival 06 - 12 – 24 (Months)		
[20]	2000	27	66	100	70	–	32	22	22
[16]	2000	17	60	98	33	18	–	56	47
[104]	1998	129	66	78	78	17	60	52	29
[21]	2001	78	–	–	23	–	65	34	–
Pooled DT MCSD estimated survival	1998–2001	251	65	90	57	<20	50	40	30
[21]	2001	655	50	81	–	–	68	55	–

Abbreviations: DT, destination therapy; IHD, ischemic heart disease; LVEF, left ventricular ejection fraction.

Data from Cadeiras M, von Bayern MP, Pal A, et al. Destination therapy: an alternative for end-stage heart failure patients not eligible for heart transplantation. Current Opinion in Organ Transplantation 2005;10:369.

Current limitations of destination mechanical circulatory support devices

Current destination mechanical circulatory support devices limitation #1: infections

Infection causes substantial morbidity and mortality after MCSD implantation and reduces the survival and QoL benefit [23–28]. As opposed to the risk of coagulopathies, which occur early after MCSD-implantation, the risk of infection increases linearly (Fig. 1) [21]. Infection can develop in the percutaneously placed drive line, the generator pocket, and the bloodstream and is often initiated by mechanical disruption of the interface between the tissue and the drive line manifested as drainage requiring antibiotics, surgical excision, or revision of the exit site. Because MCSDs are considered life sustaining, explanting or replacing the entire infected device is a risky, if not impossible, option. Infection was observed in 50% of patients bridged to transplantation with 40% being MCSD-related bloodstream infection, occurring more frequently among patients who have diabetes. The third MCSD report demonstrates that as shown in many single-center studies, infection continues to be the major complication limiting outcomes at 1 year [21]. Numerous factors predispose MCSD patients to infection including postoperative bleeding necessitating reoperation, endotracheal tubes, intravascular catheters, and other indwelling tubes necessary for the care of postsurgical patients. Control of infection may be improved with new MCSD designs, antibiotic impregnated drivelines [29], and innovative therapies such as antibiotic beads or change in the antibiotic use strategies [28].

In the bridge to transplantation experience with the MicroMed DeBakey Bridge to Transplantation trial, only few patients had device-related infection [15,30,31], suggesting that developments in the design of the device played an important role in controlling infection. Novel advances to avoid infection include the use of transcutaneous energy transmission, initially introduced in the clinical setting by the LionHeart LVAD-2000 (Arrow International, Reading, Pennsylvania), a completely implantable left ventricular assist device [32]. The preliminary experience showed no infection episodes [33] in addition to low incidence of central nervous system complications [34]. This left ventricular assist system was discontinued in 2005, before the first long-term patient support in the US was published [35].

It is clear the tremendous role that infection control plays in limiting MCSD outcomes. Therefore, the development of new strategies to study MCSD-related infection is an important goal. The authors' group at Columbia University has developed a miniaturized mice model of HeartMate I-type MCSD to resemble the left ventricular assist device (LVAD) membrane/blood interphase [36]. A homemade video of the procedure

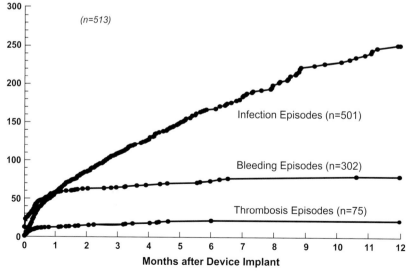

Fig. 1. Incidence of adverse events after MCSD implantation. (*Data from* Deng MC, Edwards LB, Taylor DO, et al. Mechanical circulatory support device database of the international society for heart and lung transplantation: third annual report-2005. J Heart Lung Transplant 2005;24:1182–7.)

can be accessed at the following URL address: http://cardiactransplantresearch.cumc.columbia.edu/AnimalModelsOfMechanicalSupport.htm. Using this model and a novel in vitro binding assay with VAD membranes and a heterologous lactococcal system of expression, the authors identified three S. aureus proteins–clumping factor A (ClfA) and fibronectin binding proteins A and B (FnBPA and FnBPB) as the main proteins involved in adherence to VAD polyurethane membranes. Adherence was greatly diminished by long implantation times, reflecting a change in topologic features of the VAD membrane [37]. These observations led the authors to use a synthetic peptide to interfere with these adherence mechanisms in the murine assist device model (F. Lowy, unpublished data, 2007). Driveline infections will continue to be a problem faced by most of the devices that are currently being tested in randomized clinical trials, and models for its study have also been published by the authors' center [38]. Advantages from devices used to treat infection may also be an important complement to practice. Treatment of driveline drainage benefited from vacuum-assisted closure [39], which may increase granulation tissue and reduce bacterial burden [40]. In addition, infection control will also benefit from a team trained to prevent infections. A recent randomized study showed that an evidence-based intervention resulted in 66% sustained reduction in rates of catheter-related bloodstream in patients in the intensive care unit [41].

Current destination mechanical circulatory support devices limitation #2: coagulopathies

Next to infection, coagulation problems leading to clotting–stroke limited the survival and QoL benefit from long-term mechanical support in the REMATCH experience [42]. As opposed to the risk of infection, which augments linearly after MCSD-implantation, the risk of coagulopathies including bleeding and clot-associated embolic stroke is clustered in the early postoperative period (see Fig. 1) [21]. Technologic development has lead to a significant reduction in the incidence of embolic events [43]. There is still the need to improve coagulation monitoring techniques and anticoagulation protocols and identify patients prone to development of antiplatelet resistance that might be present in more than 50% of all patients on chronic therapy with aspirin or clopidogrel [44] or differential responsiveness to anticoagulants related to specific haplotypes [45]. Severe bleeding can be difficult to control in patients who have prolonged cardiogenic shock and alteration of hepatic and renal flow with subsequent coagulopathy. Patients who have prolonged severe cardiogenic shock requiring implantation of a biventricular assist device may develop diffuse bleeding due to alteration of hepatic and renal function and subsequent coagulopathy. Recombinant activated factor VII was reported to successfully control massive bleeding after implantation of assist devices [46–50].

Current destination mechanical circulatory support devices limitation #3: right ventricular failure

Although MCSD pumping leads to a progressive decrease of pulmonary vascular resistances and normalization of pulmonary pressures, improving right ventricular performance and geometry [51,52], insertion of an implantable MCSD complicated by early right ventricular failure has a poor prognosis and remains largely unpredictable [53]. Improving evaluation of right ventricular function before insertion of an assist device and the development of less-invasive temporary implantable mechanical support, percutaneous right ventricular assist devices, and new drugs that may be used to lower right ventricular afterload may help improve outcomes in the presence of right ventricular dysfunction. The utility of clinical variables for predicting right ventricular dysfunction including preoperative low mean pulmonary artery and the impairment of hepatic and renal function has been repeatedly reported [53–56]. Future research might be necessary to identify variables that might be more sensitive of the right ventricle for patients who have or do not have similar degrees of end organ dysfunction. For example, in patients who have heart failure from left ventricular systolic dysfunction, the presence of coexistent right ventricular dysfunction may be evaluated with right ventricular myocardial performance index. Wider use of this nongeometric parameter may help to identify patients for whom options for further intervention should be carefully evaluated [57]. Improvements in right ventricular assist device support development may improve survival in these patients. Currently, clinically available right ventricular assist devices (RVADs) are extracorporeal devices and have several limitations, such as need for anticoagulation, need for hospital stay, and less than ideal QoL. The DexAide RVAD, follows the CoRAideLVD-4000 Assist System (Arrow International, Reading, Pennsylvania) design but with reduced diameter of the primary impeller blades and blade count to allow an operating speed range of 1800 to 3200 rpm, lower than that of LVAD because of the lower resistance of pulmonary circulation while maintaining reduced thrombogenicity and long durability [58]. For shorterterm support, small devices that reduce surgical damage while allowing adequate support may improve bridging to right ventricle recovery. A miniaturized rotary blood pump with a diameter of 6.4 mm and a weight of 11 g has been implanted to bypass the ventricle between the right atrium and main pulmonary artery in experimental animals. The inner volume of the pump is 12 mL, and the inner artificial blood-contacting surface is 65 cm^2. The pump consists of a rotor driven by an incorporated brushless direct current motor, the housing of the rotor, the inflow cage, the outflow cannula, and the driveline. At the maximum speed of 32,500 rotations/min, the pump can deliver a flow of 6 L/min. The initial study results with the microaxial blood pump are promising as a device for right ventricular support [59]. Developments to improve clinical management (ie, by obtaining a sustained reduction of right ventricular afterload) may facilitate weaning from inhaled nitric oxide and inotropic support minimizing deleterious hemodynamic consequences [60].

Current destination mechanical circulatory support devices limitation #4: device dysfunction

Device dysfunction not infrequently complicates follow-up (see Table 2). Within established types of MCSDs, improvements have been made to ensure better outcomes [61,62]. In a single-center report, the cumulative probability of device failure was gradually increasing up to a 64% at 2 years with major failures occurring in near 8% including vented electric failure, seized motor, rupture of pump diaphragm, inlet valve regurgitation, fracture of the power cable, and inlet valve regurgitation [63]. Technologic advances over the last decade led to refinement in design and implantation techniques of assist devices. The reliability of the two most recent design iterations of the XVE pump (stitch modification to the inflow valve assembly and new inflow valve housing redesign) was compared with the earlier VE version in 268 devices implanted in 245 patients. Significantly fewer major device malfunctions occurred within the XVE group compared with the VE group. The number of major device malfunctions per patient-year of support for inflow valve dysfunction,

bearing wear, and other failures for the VE and XVE were significantly reduced [61,62,64], although changes in the design may have also adversely affected the durability beyond the second year [65]. The durability and reliability of the Novacor assist device is well recognized [66]. First experiences with new generation devices are growing. Recently, it has been reported a patient was supported over 6 years by the Jarvik 2000 assist device [67]. The Jarvik 2000 assist device experience showed a 95% freedom from system failure at 4 years without implantable component failure with no implantable component failure. Device malfunctions were related to external cables and lack of a backup battery. Noncorrosive, gold-plated stainless steel connectors were incorporated to prevent corrosion observed on the connectors to the retroauricular power supply. The implantability and durability of this device, in addition to the exchangeability of external components, give promise for long-term circulatory support in critically ill patients who have heart failure.

Current destination mechanical circulatory support devices limitations and clinical implementation delay

Despite the first randomized clinical data showing a survival and QoL benefit, the implementation of destination therapy and adoption by the clinical community has been slower than expected. According to different experts [8,68], the reasons include concerns about long-term survival, device-related morbidity, reimbursement issues, and lack of awareness about this new treatment modality. Therefore, from November 2002, the time of FDA-approval, to November 2005, there were 311 HeartMate XVE destination therapy recipients at 65 centers in the US [69], corresponding to an annual rate of 104 implantations. Although the CMS US national coverage decision in October 2003 resulted in an increase from 3 to 11 implantations per month, the rate seems to have declined. These numbers are as much as three orders of magnitude below the original National Institutes of Health projections [70,71]. The successful implementation of destination MCSD in routine cardiovascular medicine practice will depend on progress in several areas, including patient selection and education, patient management [72], outcomes analysis resulting from multiple institutional reports, randomized clinical trials, the ISHLT MCSD database and the INTERMACS endeavor [73], and MCSD-technology development (The major experiences in clinical MCSD are summarized in Table 2, and the major characteristics of the assist device in Table 3) [12,13].

Mechanical circulatory support devices development/design and progress

In this section, the authors review current scientific evidence as it relates to MCSD-technology development and derive hypotheses for the future development of MCSD based on major areas that they found actionable for MCSD progress. In the authors' opinion, MCSD progress should be an integrated effort that originates in the clinical encounter brought to the coordinated evaluation of experts, regulatory agencies, payers, and industry and focusing in seven major areas of development including assist device size, mode of action, biocompatibility, implantability, manageability, durability, and cost (Fig. 2).

To improve understanding of the drawbacks of each technology, it is important to critically review the clinical experience with the different assist device systems. Because of the lack of consistent definitions in the reporting of MCSD-related adverse events, evaluation of event rates and endpoints, and making side-to-side comparisons is not appropriate at this moment. Hopefully the INTERMACS project will aid in answering several of these questions. Table 4 is an evaluation of the performance of each assist device in each of the main areas of assist-device development, based on the author's opinion.

Mechanical circulatory support devices size

Hypothesis 1: mechanical circulatory support devices with smaller size reduce infection/other morbidity rate

Recipients of heart-assist devices are prone to high incidence of bleeding, and thrombo-embolic and infectious complications. The occurrence of these complications is favored by systemic alterations of coagulation and fibrinolysis, inflammation, and immune responses. Reduction of pump size may help to improve outcomes in terms of morbidity including infection. Size reduction may confine surgical damage, reduce the amount of tissue injury, limit the inflammatory response, and reduce the port-of-entry for pathogens leading to a reduced probability of clinical infection and systemic activation of the inflammatory response and coagulation cascade. For a similar characteristic of the exposed surface, limitation of the blood-contacting surfaces may decrease the time of exposure of proteins from the coagulation cascade and the probability for bacteria to adhere [74].

Rotary (axial) pumps provide two different mechanisms that may protect from infection. Rotary pumps are smaller than pulsatile pumps (see Table 2), and surgical procedure is less complicated. Continuous rather than pulsatile flow pumps may have lower infection rates [15,31,75,76]. Axial flow may prevent the creation of turbulence that prone colonization by bacteria. Axial pumps such as the DeBakey-Noon [15] and the Jarvik Flowmaker [16] are smaller and therefore offer a smaller exposure area. Those that are totally implantable such as the LionHeart LVAD (Arrow International, Reading, Pennsylvania) [75] left ventricular assist system or the AbioCor (ABIOMED Inc., Danvers, Massachusetts) [61,62] may substantially decrease the risk of ventricular assist device–related infection [33,77], but they are still limited by their size to be applicable to an extended spectrum of patients. The experience with the AbioCor orthotopic completely implantable assist device system accounted a cumulative implant time of 754 days in 7 patients. The experience of this device is still limited by outcomes and body size. The body surface area range of the patients implanted with this system was 1.83 to 2.17 m^2 (see Table 2). In the authors' program, less than half of the patients that underwent transplantation between 2001 and 2005 had a surface area greater than 1.8 m^2. The LionHeart completely implantable assist device may better adjust to smaller patients. Device-related infections were compared between the HeartMate left ventricular assist device and the Jarvik 2000 permanent LVAD over a total support time of 1626 patient-days (HeartMate, 26–271 days) versus 1246 patient-days (Jarvik 2000, 8–411 days). Driveline infections resolved with antibiotics and local wound care in the Jarvik 2000 patient, but only in 1 of 7 HeartMate patients. Implantation of the Jarvik 2000 was associated with less device-related infections than the HeartMate LVAD. The power-supply of the permanent Jarvik 2000 is suitable for long-term mechanical support [16]. The experience with the InCor (Berlin Heart AG, Berlin, Germany) assist device, a small, implantable, magnetically accentuated axial flow pump, showed no early bleeding complications and an absence of device-related infections [75]. A match-controlled comparison of 50 patients with the continuous flow device Micromed (DeBakey, Houston, Texas) or InCor (Berlin Heart AG, Berlin, Germany) and the pulsatile device Novacor

Table 2

Characteristics of major experiences with mechanical circulatory support devices that underwent clinical evaluation

Study / Assist device	References	MCSD Type	Indication	Weight (grams)	LxW (mm2)	Fmax (L/min)	Study Start	Study End	Patients Total	Male	%	Fem.	%	Age Mean	Min	Max	Area Mean	Min	Max	Etiology CAD	%CAD	Time Mean	Min	Max	Total
AbioCor	[61,62]	Pulsatile	DT	—	—	—	2001	NA	7	7	100	0	0	66.7	51	79	NA	1.83	2.17	6	85.71	108	0	234	754
Arrow LionHeart	[32]	Pulsatile	DT	—	—	—	1999	2002	23	14	60.87	9	39.13	65	58	69	—	NA	—	14	60.87	347	17	1259	7980
Berlin Heart InCor	[75]	Axial Flow	BTT	200	3600	7	—	2004	15	10	66.67	5	33.33	45	24	59	1.89	1.63	2.28	9	60	132	9	436	2265
HeartMate I	[94]	Pulsatile	BTT	1000	6496	10	1993	1997	32	26	81.25	6	18.75	49	11	65	—	—	—	18	56.25	122	3	605	2140
HeartMate I	[95]	Pulsatile	BTT			10	1991	1996	97	—	—	—	—	53.9	27	70	—	—	—	67	69.07	70	—	206	6790
HeartMate I	[105]	Pulsatile	BTT			10	1993	1997	16	10	62.5	6	37.5	46	16	63	1.9	1.6	2.4	2	12.5	140	54	310	2644
HeartMate I	[106]	Pulsatile	BTT			10	1992	1998	114	98	85.96	16	14.04	46	11	64	—	—	—	23	20.18	50	6	184	4818
HeartMate I	[107]	Pulsatile	BTT			10	1996	1998	280	232	82.86	48	17.14	55	21	67	1.97	1.45	2.75	149	53.21	112	1	691	31390
HeartMate I	[9]	Pulsatile	DT			10	1998	2001	68	53	77.94	15	22.06	66	NA	NA	—	—	—	53	77.94	408	NA	—	24929
HeartMate I	[108]	Pulsatile	BTT			10	1996	2004	119	104	87.39	15	12.61	52	NA	NA	—	NA	—	49	41.18	71	0	448	8449
HeartMate I	[43]	Pulsatile	BTT			10	1999	2002	51	42	82.35	9	17.65	54.4	NA	NA	—	NA	—	27	52.94	138	NA	—	7038
HeartMate II	[109]	Axial Flow	BTT/DT	396	2800	10.5	2005	2006	15	11	73.33	4	26.67	40	14	65	—	NA	—	4	26.67	178	6	693	2663
Jarvik FlowMaker	[16]	Axial Flow	DT	90	1375	6	2000	2004	17	16	94.12	1	5.882	60	49	74	2	1.5	2.3	4	23.53	293	30	528	5996
Jarvik FlowMaker	[110]	Axial Flow	BTT/DT	—	—	6	2000	2004	102	—	NA	—		—	NA		—	NA		—	NA	212	NA	1788	21535
Jarvik7 (CardioWest)	[111]	Pulsatile	BTT	—	—	—	1986	2001	127	108	85.04	19	14.96	38	11	64	1.81	1.37	NA	38	29.92	NA	0	602	3606
Micromed DeBakey	[31]	Axial Flow	BTT	114	2318	10	1998	2002	150	123	82	27	18	48	12	73	1.8	1.4	2.34	—	NA	75	NA	441	11096
Micromed DeBakey	[15]	Axial Flow	BTT			10	—	NA	30	20	66.67	10	33.33	53	20	69	1.9	1.3	2.3	17	56.67	42	9	111	1260
Micromed DeBakey	[30]	Axial Flow	BTT			10	2002	2004	17	12	70.59	5	29.41	44	NA	—	1.7	NA	—	5	29.41	90.3	11	443	1503
Novacor LVAS	[43]	Pulsatile	BTT	1000	21780	12	1999	2002	13	12	92.31	1	7.692	51.6	NA	—	—	NA	—	8	61.54	114	NA	—	1482
Novacor LVAS	[112]	Pulsatile	BTT			12	1993	1999	464	413	89.01	51	10.99	49	16	75	1.92	1.39	2.68	124	26.72	100	0	1477	65335
Novacor LVAS (ePTFE)	[66]	Pulsatile	NA			12	1998	2000	88	—	NA	—		51	14	68	—	NA	—	77	87.5	120	0	921	10620
Novacor LVAS (Pol)	[113]	Pulsatile	BTT			12	1996	1999	282	237	84.04	45	15.96	48.1	NA	—	1.94	NA	—	118	41.84	97	NA	—	27936
Novacor LVAS (Vasc)	[113]	Pulsatile	BTT			12	1996	1999	202	166	82.18	36	17.82	48.7	NA	—	1.94	NA	—	80	39.6	91	NA	—	18382
CardioWest TAH	[114]	Pulsatile	BTT	160		9.5	1992	2002	81	70	86.42	11	13.58	51	NA	—	2	NA	—	53	65.43	79.1	NA	—	6407
CardioWest TAH	[115]	Pulsatile	BTT			9.5	2001	2003	42	37	88.1	5	11.9	51	15	74	1.9	1.5	2.4	20	47.62	86	1	291	3612
Totals	25	—	—	—	—	9.9	1986	2006	2445	1814	80.08	344	19.92	50.7	11	75	1.9	1.3	2.75	43.6	47.3	138	0	1788	279876

Study		MCSD		Infection			Bleeding			Neurological			Dysfunction			Outcomes									
Assist device	References	Type	Indication	N	%	Incid	N	%	Incid	N	%	Incid	N	%	Incid	BTT	%	Wean	%	Mort	%	Incid	1 year	TxSv	%
AbioCor	[61,62]	Pulsatile	DT	0	0	0	4	57.1	1.94	3	42.86	1.45	0	0	0.00	0	0	0	0	5	71.43	2.42	—	NA	—
Arrow LionHeart	[32]	Pulsatile	DT	— NA —			— NA —			57	247.8	2.61	— NA —			— NA —		NA		6	40	0.967	—	NA	—
Berlin Heart InCor	[75]	Flow	BTT	0	0		—	—		4	26.67	0.64	3	20	0.48	5	33.33	1	6.667	6	18.75	1.023	—	NA	—
HeartMate I	[94]	Pulsatile	BTT	8	25	1.36	4	26.7	0.64	4	6.25	0.34	3	20	0.51	20	62.5	1	3.125	24	24.74	1.29	69	NA	93.2
Heartmate I	[95]	Pulsatile	BTT	57	58.8	3.06	4	12.5	0.68	2	6.25	0.11	12	9.38	0.65	74	76.29	2	2.062	1	6.25	0.138	7	NA	58.3
HeartMate I	[105]	Pulsatile	BTT	10	62.5	1.38	20	20.6	1.08	2	2.062	0.28	20	12.4	2.76	12	75	1	6.25	34	29.82	2.576	—	NA	—
HeartMate I	[106]	Pulsatile	BTT	41	36	1.45	6	37.5	0.83	16	12.5	1.21	4	3.51	0.30	57	50	3	2.632	82	29.29	0.953	158	NA	84
HeartMate I	[107]	Pulsatile	BTT	125	44.6	1.24	28	24.6	2.12	75	14.04	0.87	3	1.07	0.03	188	67.14	10	3.571	41	60.29	0.6	—	NA	—
HeartMate I	[9]	Pulsatile	DT	— NA —			31	11.1	0.36		26.79	0.39				0	0	0	0	20	16.81	0.864	—	NA	—
HeartMate I	[108]	Pulsatile	BTT	15	29.4	0.78	— NA —			1	1.961	0.05	5	9.8	0.26	88	73.95	0	0	15	29.41	0.778	78	NA	88.6
HeartMate I	[43]	Pulsatile	BTT	— NA —			— NA —				6.667	0.14		6.67	0.14	36	70.59	0	0	2	13.33	0.274	31	NA	86.1
HeartMate II	[109]	Flow	BTT/DT	1	5.88	0.06	1	5.88	0.06	4	23.53	0.24				1	6.667	0	0	8	47.06	0.487	—	NA	—
Jarvik FlowMaker	[16]	Flow	DT	— NA —			— NA —			— NA —			10	9.8	0.17	1	5.882	0	0	—	—		—	NA	—
Jarvik FlowMaker	[110]	Flow	BTT/DT	4	3.15	0.40	33	26	3.34	2	1.575	0.20	1	0.79	0.10	— NA —		NA		—	—		—	NA	—
(CardioWest)	[111]	Pulsatile	BTT	5	3.33	0.16	48	32	1.58	16	10.67	0.53	4	2.67	0.13	62	41.33	1	0.667	68	45.33	2.237	7	NA	77.8
Micromed DeBakey	[31]	Flow	BTT	2	6.67	0.58	8	26.7	2.32	3	10	0.87	0	0	0.00	20	66.67	0	0	0	0	0	—	NA	—
Micromed DeBakey	[15]	Flow	BTT	0	0	0.00	4	23.5	0.97	3	11.76	0.49	0	0	0.00	14	82.35	0	0	2	11.76	0.486	—	NA	—
Micromed DeBakey	[30]	Flow	BTT	5	38.5	1.23	— NA —			3	23.08	0.74	0	0	0.00	9	69.23	0	0	2	15.38	0.493	—	NA	—
Novacor LVAS	[43]	Pulsatile	BTT	— NA —			59	12.7	0.33	— NA —			0	0	0.00	155	33.41	21	4.526	147	31.68	0.821	—	NA	—
Novacor LVAS	[112]	Pulsatile	BTT	— NA —			— NA —			9	10.23	0.31	— NA —			— NA —		NA		—	—		—	NA	—
(ePTFE)	[65]	Pulsatile	NA	— NA —			— NA —						— NA —			— NA —				—	—		—	NA	—
Novacor LVAS (Pol)	[113]	Pulsatile	BTT	104	36.9	1.36	82	29.1	1.07	54	19.15	0.71	— NA —			— NA —		NA		82	29.08	1.071	—	NA	—
(Vasc)	[113]	Pulsatile	BTT	58	28.7	1.15	59	29.2	1.17	23	11.39	0.46	— NA —			— NA —				65	32.18	1.291	—	NA	—
CardioWest TAH	[114]	Pulsatile	BTT	29	35.8	1.65	23	28.4	1.31	5	6.173	0.28	1	1.23	0.06	64	79.01	0	0	17	20.99	0.968	55	NA	85.9
CardioWest TAH	[115]	Pulsatile	BTT	5	11.9	0.51	8	19	0.81	4	9.524	0.40	2	4.76	0.20	11	26.19	0	0	24	57.14	2.425	—	NA	—
Totals	25			26.1	23.7	1.03	24.8	24.9	1.18	13.7	24.98	0.61	3.6	10.9	0.29	45.39	51.09	2.22	1.639	32.3	27.97		57.9	—	82

Because of differences in adverse event reporting criteria, data might be incomplete or interpreted differently and not accurately comparable for the experiences with different assist devices. For an in-deep analysis, the authors suggest readers to refer to the original publication.

Abbreviations: DT, destination therapy; ePTFE, expanded polytetrafluoroethylene; LVAS, left ventricular assist system; TAH, total artificial heart.

Table 3
Characteristics of currently available mechanical circulatory support devices

Type	Ventricle	Flow	Pump position	Implant #
AbioCor	Total heart	Pulsatile	Intrathoracic	>10
Abiomed	Left & right	Pulsatile	Paracorporeal	>3000
Berlin Heart InCor	Left	Nonpulsatile	Intra-abdominal	>250
Berlin Heart EXCOR	Left & right	Pulsatile	Paracorporeal	>30
CardioWest	Total heart	Pulsatile	Intrathoracic	>200
CorAide (Terumo)	Left	Nonpulsatile	Intra-abdominal	>2
DuraHeart (Terumo)	Left	Nonpulsatile	Intra-abdominal	preclinical
EVAHEART	Left	Nonpulsatile	Intra-abdominal	preclinical
HeartWare	Left	Nonpulsatile	Intra-abdominal	1
Jarvik 2000	Left	Nonpulsatile	Intra-abdominal	>100
Lionheart	Left	Pulsatile	Intra-addominal	>25
Medos	Left & right	Pulsatile	Paracorporeal	>200
Micromed-DeBakey	Left	Nonpulsatile	Intra-abdominal	>380
Thoratec HeartMate	Left	Pulsatile	Intra-abdominal	>4100
Thoratec HeartMate II	Left	Nonpulsatile	Intra-abdominal	>50
Thoratec HeartMate III	Left	Nonpulsatile	Intra-abdominal	Preclinical
Thoratec TLC II	Left & right	Pulsatile	Paracorporeal	>2800
Thoratec iVAD	Left & right	Pulsatile	Intra-abdominal	>30
Ventracor	Left	Nonpulsatile	Intra-abdominal	>60
Worldheart Novacor	Left	Pulsatile	Intra-abdominal	>1700
Worldheart Novacor Rotary	Left	Nonpulsatile	Intra-abdominal	>1
Worldheart Novacor II	Left	Pulsatile	Intra-abdominal	Preclinical

Data from Deng MC, Naka Y. Mechanical circulatory support therapy in advanced heart failure. London: Imperial College Press; 2007.

(WorldHeart, Oakland, California) or HeartMate (Thoratec Corp, Pleasanton, California) showed similar rates of successful bridging to transplantation and long-term survival after transplantation and cause of death [78].

Hypothesis 2: mechanical circulatory support devices with smaller size increase patient spectrum

Body size is not an uncommon concern in patients undergoing MCSD implantation. In the authors' program at Columbia University, near 20% of the patients that underwent heart transplantation between 2001 and 2005 had a body surface area lower than $1.5 \, m^2$. The introduction of assist devices for these patients has been recently accomplished, and use of assist devices beyond ECMO was successful even in the pediatric population. Children underwent mechanical circulatory support implantation operation with Thoratec LVAD, biventricular Thoratec VAD, the Medos-HIA system (Helmholtz Institute, Aachen, Germany), Berlin Heart Excor System, and the Novacor LVAD. The indication in these patients was bridge to transplantation. The incidence of complications including bleeding, thrombosis, infection, and neurologic events was elevated while intracorporeal implantation was unlikely, at least

in the infant [79–81]. In the US, the DeBakey assist device has gained FDA approval to be used in the pediatric population. To develop smaller size pumps suitable to pediatric candidates, the National Heart, Lung, and Blood Institute awarded five contracts to develop a family of devices that includes an implantable mixed-flow ventricular assist device designed specifically for patients up to 2 years of age, another mixed-flow ventricular assist device that can be implanted intravascularly or extravascularly depending on patient size, a compact integrated pediatric cardiopulmonary assist system, an apically implanted axial-flow ventricular assist device, and a pulsatile-flow ventricular assist device; to reliably provide circulatory support for infants and children while minimizing risks related to infection, bleeding, and thromboembolism [82].

Mechanical circulatory support devices mode of action

Hypothesis 3: pulsatile axial flow mechanical circulatory support devices may improve outcomes

Although it has been proposed that change in the circulatory physiology from a pulsatile to a nonpulsatile irrigation system may be deleterious (ie, by preventing from retrograding multiple

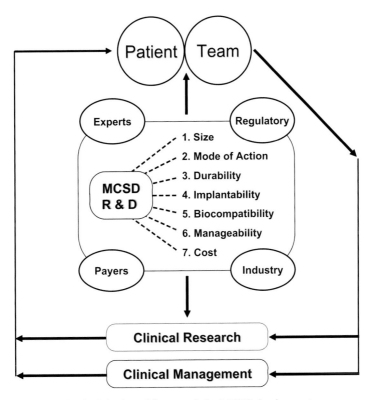

Fig. 2. Criteria and framework for MCSD development.

organ failure or causing less systemic inflammation), it has not been demonstrated whether this would translate into a significant difference in clinical outcomes (see Table 2) [15,16,21,71,75,83]. Both types of devices can achieve a similar degree of left ventricular pressure unloading, but ventricular volume unloading was less pronounced with the continuous flow devices [83,84]. In both types of devices, there was an equivalent reduction in cellular markers of myocardial failure/overload including myocardial tumor necrosis factor-α, total collagen, and mycocyte size [84], suggesting a beneficial effect on the ultrastructural architecture of the failing heart. It has been proposed that nonpulsatile perfusion does not have any negative effects on capillary perfusion during chronic support, because of absence of pulsatility at this level, but pulsatility does exist in capillaries that significantly improve the velocity of erythrocytes at the capillary level. Because the natural heart is also contracting, arterial waveforms show some degree of pulsatility [85]. The real effect of pulsatility and nonpulsatility in the chronic setting of MCSD is still poorly understood. A challenging development in MCSD technology is the

combination of both modalities, therefore gaining the efficiency of the axial flow while conserving the physiology and clinical benefits—if any—of the pulsatile flow. Animal experiments with the continuous flow, centrifugal pump Thoratec Heart-Mate III (Thoratec, Burlington, Massachusetts) were done to achieve LVAD-induced pulsatile flow by sharply alternating the speed of the magnetically levitated rotor of the left pump during the artificial diastole and systole, setting a device rate and a systolic interval within the normal physiologic ranges. To achieve this goal of simulating a pulsatile circulation, it required high technologic advances including stiff speed control, low rotor mass, and robust magnetic rotor suspension that resulted in a responsive system that enabled rapid speed changes [86].

Mechanical circulatory support devices durability

Hypothesis 4: mechanical circulatory support devices with higher durability decrease mortality and morbidity

There is currently no randomized comparison on the durability of assist device and overall

Table 4
Characteristics of currently available mechanical circulatory support device within the framework of the "ideal mechanical circulatory support device design"

Type	Size reduction	Durability	Implantability	Biocompatibility	Cost	Manageability
Ideal Future MCSD	+++	+++	+++	+++	+++	+++
AbioCor	+	—	+++	—	+	+
Abiomed	—	—	—	—	—	—
Berlin Heart InCor	+++	+++	+	—	+	++
CardioWest	+	++	+	—	+	+
CorAide	++	—	—	—	—	—
EVAHEART	+	—	—	—	—	—
Jarvik 2000	++	+++	+	—	+	++
Lionheart	+	—	+++	—	+	+
Medos	—	+	—	—	—	—
Micromed-DeBakey	++	—	—	—	—	—
Terumo Duraheart	++	—	+	—	—	—
Thoratec HeartMate	+	+	+	++	+	+
Thoratec HeartMate II	++	—	—	—	—	—
Thoratec	—	—	—	—	—	—
Ventracor	++	—	+	—	+	+
Worldheart Novacor	—	+++	—	+	+	+
Novacor II	+++	+++	+++	+	+	++

Data from Deng MC, Naka Y. Mechanical circulatory support therapy in advanced heart failure. London: Imperial College Press; 2007.

mortality. Data from published experiences do not clearly support the hypothesis that mortality or transplantation rates might be lower in patients receiving assist devices with higher durability, mostly because the experiences in MCSD as destination therapy is limited. Only isolated reports suggested uninterrupted MCSD support during more than 5 years with pulsatile [70] or continuous flow [67] assist device. Long-term outcome with assist devices relies on patient selection, timing of intervention, and mechanical performance of the device. Despite efforts to improve durability of assist devices for patients undergoing destination therapy, it is most likely that MCSD recipients require exchange of the device. In the REMATCH study, 10% of the patients died due to failure of the assist device after 408 median survival days. No devices failed after 12 months, but failure rapidly increased to 35% at 24 months with 10 patients requiring replacement (see Table 2) [9]. Although multiple device replacements could be successfully performed in a single patient [87], this procedure carries higher morbidity, mortality and cost, which may hold a nonlinear relation with the risk of the first and therefore should be confined to highly selected patients. In a second attempt for implantation of an assist device, the equation will not only weigh the effect of the inflammatory response of end-stage heart failure but also the chronic activation of the inflammatory cascade, explantation of the dysfunctioning device, and implantation of the new system that may also require more prolonged surgical times. The activation of the inflammatory response after device implantation follows a well design slope that is at its maximum during the first days post MCSD, which include mediators of the innate and adaptive immunity [88]. With the growth of destination therapy as an option for MCSD recipients, patients are supported for longer periods. Using devices with higher durability that avoid the necessity of reoperation may reduce morbidity and mortality in these patients.

Hypothesis 5: mechanical circulatory support devices with higher durability decrease costs

Device failure is a limitation of permanent mechanical circulatory support and a significant economical burden of the cost of MCSD support in the long term (see Table 2). It is related to long admissions, and device exchange by itself is complication prone. The mechanical reliability of the Jarvik 2000 assist device, the DeBakey-Noon device as well as the Novacor Assist System is encouraging. The experience with the Jarvik 2000 assist device in more than 100 patients implanted either as a bridge-to-transplantation or as lifetime therapy found no implantable component failure in vivo and during bench testing after a cumulative pump run-time of 110 years, 59 years overall in vivo and 51 years in vitro. In a recent report it was shown that the cost of device therapy practice was lowered since the REMATCH study was published [89], but still, an economic evaluation that summarized the available evidence in MCSD costs has shown that neither LVAD indication is a cost-effective use. For the HeartMate LVAD used as a BTT, the cost per quality adjusted life year (QALY) was £65,242 (~US$125,300). In the less-restrictive indication, destination therapy was not cost-effective. The baseline cost per QALY of the first-generation HeartMate LVAD was £170,616 (~US$327,900), whereas the hypothetical scenario based on the cost of the second-generation MicroMed DeBakey device illustrated that a 60% improvement in survival over first-generation devices was necessary before the incremental cost-effectiveness approached £40,000 (~US$76,900) per QALY [90]. From the LVAD population at Columbia Presbyterian Medical Center, discharged following HeartMate vented electric implantation, the mean pre-LVAD implantation length of stay was 21.3 days, and post-LVAD length of stay was 36.8 days. Total actual hospital cost post-LVAD averaged US $197,957, and the average length of stay during a readmission was 5.6 days [91]. Most of the cost related to this type of therapy was attributable to the VAD implant and the initial hospital stay in the intensive care unit and ward [92]. LVAD complication, explantation, and implantation are associated with longer length of stay and higher cost for hospitalization.

An increase in the number of patients rather than the duration of assist device support may maintain the cost stable or higher, whereas prolongation of support with reduced cost per QALY may increase the probability of reimbursement while avoiding cost of readmissions related to device dysfunction and exchange.

Mechanical circulatory support devices—implantability

Hypothesis 6: implantable mechanical circulatory support devices decrease infection rate

Infection remains as the most common complication at limiting long-term MCSD survival (see Table 2). The probability of an organism in the bloodstream attaching to the ventricular assist device and causing ventricular assist device–related endocarditis depends on several factors, including characteristics of the device surface, the amount of turbulent blood flow in the device, and the adherence properties of the organism. For ventricular assist devices that have drivelines, host tissues and the ventricular assist device are exposed to the external contaminated environment and are often associated with other infections of the ventricular assist device and bloodstream [38]. Pumps that can be completely implanted in the thoracic cavity do not violate the abdominal anatomy, which can generate additional damage and respiratory workload during the early postoperative period. Limiting extension of the surgical insult may lead to reduction in the risk of respiratory complications [93,94].

The Arrow LionHeart LVAD 2000 left ventricular assist device was the first fully implantable system designed for destination therapy with transcutaneous energy transmission. The 2-year experience with this device in six male patients that were ineligible for heart transplantation extended over 4.5 cumulative years, with a survival rate of 50% after 18 months. There were no device-related infections. The size of the device was a limiting factor for candidate selection [33]. The AbioCor orthotopic implantable replacement heart system is powered through transcutaneous energy transfer. This device was implanted in seven patients with two early and three late deaths. No infections have been observed in this experience [61,62].

Newer generation devices, which use continuous flow technology and therefore are smaller in size, may address several of the shortcomings. Their size allows for a simpler implantation procedure, which could reduce surgical morbidity [12]. The development of transcutaneous energy supply systems is positioned as a promising solution for infection control, but it is still a challenge for device size reduction. The fully implantable system (LionHeart) reduced significantly the system-related infection complications. Further miniaturization of the systems might reduce the comorbidities and increase the acceptance of this therapeutic option in the management of end-stage cardiac failure [33].

Hypothesis 7: implantable mechanical circulatory support devices improve quality of life

Implantable MCSD allowed for patient discharge during short periods [95,96]. Outpatient management after LVAD implantation became feasible, while severe complications were uncommon [97]. The implementation of an out-of-hospital management option has led to a significant

improvement in the quality of life of those patients. However, assist devices are still associated
with a considerable number of complications.
The different devices differ in terms of location,
type of support, and driving units. They are suitable for different patients and their therapeutics
objectives. A specific protocol for selection and
management of patients and devices may improve
outcomes by candidacy allocation. The indication
spectrum for MCSD includes cardiogenic shock
secondary to acute myocarditis, right heart failure, acute rejection and postcardiotomy heart failure, alternative to transplantation, and bridge to
recovery. The extracorporeal devices (ie, Biomedi-
cus, Abiomed) are used for short-term support.
The Thoratec VAD and the Medos HIA-VAD
located in paracorporeal position are preferably
used for midterm support and the Novacor left
ventricular assist system (LVAS), and HeartMate
are partially implantable systems used for long-
term ventricular assistance in patients who did
not require biventricular support. Implantable devices allow discharging patients under support if
they fulfill special criteria before being discharged
to home. Careful postoperative patient management does not exclude various complications
that may vary among different devices and the patients' preoperative conditions [98]. Continuous
flow blood pumps provided symptomatic relief
of severe heart failure with high quality of life
scores [16].

*Mechanical circulatory support
devices—biocompatibility*

*Hypothesis 8: biocompatible mechanical
circulatory support devices reduce adverse events*

   Neurologic events such as thromboembolic
and hemorrhagic strokes are common complications of mechanical circulatory support (see Table 2). A prospective single-center study compared
the safety and effectiveness of the Novacor (Novacor N100) left ventricular assist system
(Baxter Health care Corporation, Berkeley, California) and the HeartMate device. Neurologic
complications occurred significantly more often
among the Novacor group [99]. A change in
the material used in the inflow conduit was introduced in the late 1990s migrating from the
polyester inflow conduits (Vascutek and Cooley)
to an expanded polytetrafluoroethylene (ePTFE)
conduit. This development was based on the observation of the use of this material in vascular

grafts, proven for venous application with less
thrombogenic properties, platelet and complement activation. The outcome of this implementation was retrospectively evaluated in 310
patients receiving polyester conduits and 88 patients receiving the expanded polytetrafluoroethylene conduit. The linearized incidence of
embolic cerebrovascular accident E group was
reduced by near 50%. In animal models, biocompatible textured polyurethane is suggestive
of reduced Staphylococcal infection rates
[37,100]. Improvements in assist device development in one area may unfold new limitations
that require further exploration. For example,
the experience with continuous flow devices
compared with pulsatile devices showed an increased risk of rejection after heart transplantation [83].

*Mechanical circulatory support
devices—manageability*

*Hypothesis 9: simpler mechanical circulatory
support devices decrease mortality and morbidity*

   Although implantable left ventricular assist
devices have been remarkably free of mechanical
failures, uncommon malfunctions that are related
to manageability may have dramatic outcomes.
The Novacor N100 PCq LVAS was susceptible to
internal short circuit of the device due to urine aspiration by way of the vent line. This scenario required device replacement [101]. A similar event
was also described for the HeartMate MCSD.
Fluid was aspirated into the vent port, resulting
in the malfunction of the device and a clinical
emergency [102]. The SynCardia CardioWest total
artificial heart SynCardia Systems Inc., Tucson,
Arizona is a biventricular, orthotopic, pneumatic,
pulsatile blood pump driven by an external con-
sole. In a single-center experience with this device
in 62 patients, 2 out of 10 patients died because of
catheter entrapment in the tricuspid valve. The
AbioCor technology incorporates a radiofre-
quency transmitter, which sends information
from the internal controller to the external con-
sole which includes among others, a continuous
real-time telemetry of hydraulic pressure waveforms [61,62] that may in the future avoid this
type of complication while having closer follow-
up of the patient. The development of assist devices should also contemplate common activities
of daily activity that may compromise their
functioning.

Mechanical circulatory support devices—cost

Hypothesis 10: simpler and less expensive mechanical circulatory support devices increase insurance coverage rate and population distribution

Serious LVAD-related complications may negate the benefits of LVAD implantation, resulting in increased costs associated with implantation. Infection is the most frequent complication during long-term MCSD support. Prevention of device-related infection is crucial to the cost-effective use of mechanical circulatory support devices. Adherence to evidence-based infection control and prevention guidelines, meticulous surgical technique, and optimal postoperative surgical site care form the foundation for LVAD-associated infection [103]. A retrospective analysis done in patients who had a HeartMate XVE pump implanted as destination therapy at two high-volume ventricular assist device implant centers after US FDA approval in the post-REMATCH era showed 40% lower mean hospital costs when measured from implantation to discharge [89], which was naturally bounded to an increase coverage decision. Reducing costs should increase coverage and reimbursement ranges as the number of implants increase. For example, the United Kingdom Department of Health allocates funds for ventricular assist device implantation as a bridge to transplantation at three centers. The cost-effectiveness of this program showed that mean quality-adjusted life-years for an assist-device patient was 3.27 at a lifetime cost of US$316,078, whereas inotrope-dependent transplant candidates had mean quality-adjusted life-years of 4.99 at a lifetime cost of US$238,011. Patients undergoing assist-device implantation had significant quality-adjusted life-years, but more expensive than the worst conventional clinical scenario [92]. Reduction in device cost to ideally reach that of routine clinical management should also lead to improvement in the coverage/reimbursement decision-making by health care programs in a proportional magnitude to the added improvement and consequently impact on the extent of the population that may get benefit from this device. Simpler MCSD may also increase insurance coverage rate and population distribution. Nonpulsatile LVAD recipients had a significantly smaller body surface area, required shorter cardiopulmonary bypass time, and reduced initial intensive care unit stay without affecting difference in post-LVAD outcomes [71]. For similarly ill patients congestive heart failure, nonpulsatile LVAD provided comparable benefit in patients with reduced by-pass time and reduced initial intensive care unit stay, therefore indicating simplicity of implantation, reduced cost, and applicability to a wider range of recipients. Optimizing efforts in identifying a device that would suit the vast majority of the patients that is durable and easy to implant may reduce the gap between coverage and population distribution.

Summary

The new generation of assist devices should be capable of mimicking as many of the native heart pump attributes restoring normal function and minimizing acute and chronic damage in the interphase of each of its components and the human body and of the human body and the assist device MCSD technology. Improvement along the lines of the outlined criteria will broaden the use of this technology. For this to occur, fundamental engineering challenges related to (1) size, (2) mode of action, (3) durability, (4) implantability, (5) biocompatibility, (6) manageability, and (7) cost should be overcome. Physiologically adaptive implantable heart pumps would ideally improve prolonged chronic mechanical circulatory support, while reducing costs will make this therapy more widely affordable while demonstrating improved clinical outcomes, better quality of life that will also improve future cost–utility analyses.

References

[1] Bardy GH, Lee KL, Mark DB, et al. Sudden Cardiac Death in Heart Failure Trial (SCD-HeFT) Investigators. Amiodarone or an implantable cardioverter-defibrillator for congestive heart failure. N Engl J Med 2005;352:225–37.

[2] Cleland JG, Daubert JC, Erdmann E, et al. Cardiac Resynchronization-Heart Failure (CARE-HF) Study Investigators. The effect of cardiac resynchronization on morbidity and mortality in heart failure. N Engl J Med 2005;352:1539–49.

[3] Crespo Leiro MG, Paniagua Martin MJ. Management of advanced or refractory heart failure. Rev Esp Cardiol 2004;57:869–83.

[4] Jimenez J, Bennett Edwards L, et al. Should stable UNOS status 2 patients be transplanted? J Heart Lung Transplant 2005;24:178–83.

[5] Juurlink DN, Mamdani MM, Lee DS, et al. Rates of hyperkalemia after publication of the Randomized Aldactone Evaluation Study. N Engl J Med 2004;351:543–51.

[6] McMurray JJ, Pfeffer MA. Heart failure. Lancet 2005;365:1877–89.

[7] Nieminen MS, Bohm M, Cowie MR, et al. Executive summary of the guidelines on the diagnosis and treatment of acute heart failure: the Task Force on Acute Heart Failure of the European Society of Cardiology. Eur Heart J 2005;26:384–416.

[8] Portner PM. The state of destination therapy for the treatment of congestive heart failure. Curr Opin Organ transplant 2006;11:546–52.

[9] Rose EA, Gelijns AC, Moskowitz AJ, et al. Long-term mechanical left ventricular assistance for end-stage heart failure. N Engl J Med 2001;345:1435–43.

[10] Park SJ, Tector A, Piccioni W, et al. Left ventricular assist devices as destination therapy: a new look at survival. J Thorac Cardiovasc Surg 2005;129: 9–17.

[11] Stevenson LW. Left ventricular assist devices as destination therapy for end-stage heart failure. Curr Treat Options Cardiovasc Med 2004;6:471–9.

[12] Parides MK, Moskowitz AJ, Ascheim DD, et al. Progress versus precision: challenges in clinical trial design for left ventricular assist devices. Ann Thorac Surg 2006;82(3):1140–6.

[13] Chen E, Sapirstein W, Ahn C, et al. FDA perspective on clinical trial design for cardiovascular devices. Ann Thorac Surg 2006;82(3):773–5.

[14] Available at: http://www.intermacs.org. Accessed February 22, 2007.

[15] Goldstein DJ, Zucker M, Arroyo L, et al. Safety and feasibility trial of the MicroMed DeBakey ventricular assist device as a bridge to transplantation. J Am Coll Cardiol 2005;45(6):962–3.

[16] Siegenthaler MP, Westaby S, Frazier OH, et al. Advanced heart failure: study feasibility of long term continuous axial flow pump support. Eur Heart J 2005;26:1031–8.

[17] Westaby S, Banning AP, Saito S, et al. Circulatory support for long-term treatment of heart failure: experience with an intraventricular continuous flow pump. Circulation 2002;105:2588–91.

[18] Esmore DS, Kaye D, Salamonsen R, et al. First clinical implant of the VentrAssist left ventricular assist system as destination therapy for end-stage heart failure. J Heart Lung Transplant 2005;24: 1150–4.

[19] Young JB, Rogers JG, Portner PE al. Bridge to eligibility: LVAS-support in patients with relative contraindications to transplantation. J Heart Lung Transplant 2005;24:S75.

[20] Jurmann MJ, Weng Y, Drews T, et al. Permanent mechanical circulatory support in patients of advanced age. Eur J Cardiothorac Surg 2004;25: 610–8.

[21] Deng MC, Edwards LB, Taylor DO, et al. Mechanical circulatory support device database of the international society for heart and lung transplantation: third annual report-2005. J Heart Lung Transplant 2005;24:1182–7.

[22] Deng MC, Erren M, Tjan TD, et al. Left ventricular assist system support is associated with persistent inflammation and temporary immunosuppression. Thorac Cardiovasc Surg 1999; 47(Suppl 2):326–31.

[23] Holman WL, Park SJ, Long JW, et al. Infection in permanent circulatory support: experience from the REMATCH trial. J Heart Lung Transplant 2004;23:1359–65.

[24] Horton SC, Khodaverdian R, Chatelain P, et al. Left ventricular assist device malfunction: an approach to diagnosis by echocardiography. J Am Coll Cardiol 2005;45:1435–40.

[25] Horton SC, Khodaverdian R, Powers A, et al. Left ventricular assist device malfunction: a systematic approach to diagnosis. J Am Coll Cardiol 2005; 43:1574–83.

[26] Houel R, Mazoyer E, Boval B, et al. Platelet activation and aggregation profile in prolonged external ventricular support. J Thorac Cardiovasc Surg 2004;128:197–202.

[27] Available at: http://www.jcaho.org. Accessed July 15, 2005.

[28] Simon D, Fischer S, Grossman A, et al. Left ventricular assist device-related infection: treatment and outcome. Clin Infect Dis 2005;40: 1108–15.

[29] Choi L, Choudhri AF, Pillarisetty VG, et al. Development of an infection-resistant LVAD driveline: a novel approach to the prevention of device-related infections. J Heart Lung Transplant 1999; 18(11):1103–10.

[30] Bruschi G, Ribera E, Lanfranconi M, et al. Bridge to transplantation with the MicroMed DeBakey ventricular assist device axial pump: a single centre report. J Cardiovasc Med (Hagerstown) 2006;7(2): 114–8.

[31] Goldstein DJ. Worldwide experience with MicroMed DeBakey Ventricular Assist Device as a bridge to transplantation. Circulation 2003; 108(Suppl 1):272–7.

[32] Mehta SM, Pae WE Jr, Rosenberg G, et al. The LionHeart LVD-2000: a completely implanted left ventricular assist device for chronic circulatory support. Ann Thorac Surg 2001;71(3 Suppl):S156–61; [discussion: S183–4].

[33] El-Banayosy A, Arusoglu L, Kizner L, et al. Preliminary experience with the LionHeart left ventricular assist device in patients with end-stage heart failure. Ann Thorac Surg 2003;75: 1469–75.

[34] Pae WE, Connell JM, Boehmer JP, et al. CUBS Study Group. Neurologic events with a totally implantable left ventricular assist device: European Lionheart Clinical Utility Baseline Study (CUBS). J Heart Lung Transplant 2007;26:1–8.

[35] Mehta SM, Silber D, Boehmer JP, et al. Report of the first U.S. patient successfully supported long term with the LionHeart completely implantable

left ventricular assist device system. ASAIO J 2006; 52(6):e31–2.

[36] Asai T, Baron HM, von Bayern MP, et al. A mouse aortic patch model for mechanical circulatory support. J Heart Lung Transplant 2005;24(8): 1129–32.

[37] Arrecubieta C, Asai T, Bayern M, et al. The role of Staphylococcus aureus adhesins in the pathogenesis of ventricular assist device-related infections. J Infect Dis 2006;193(8):1109–19.

[38] Sun BC, Catanese KA, Spanier TB, et al. 100 long-term implantable left ventricular assist devices: the Columbia Presbyterian interim experience. Ann Thorac Surg 1999;68(2):688–94.

[39] Yuh DD, Albaugh M, Ullrich S, et al. Treatment of ventricular assist device driveline infection with vacuum-assisted closure system. Ann Thorac Surg 2005;80(4):1493–5.

[40] Baradarian S, Stahovich M, Krause S, et al. Case series: clinical management of persistent mechanical assist device driveline drainage using vacuum-assisted closure therapy. ASAIO J 2006;52(3): 354–6.

[41] Pronovost P, Needham D, Berenholtz S, et al. An intervention to decrease catheter-related bloodstream infections in the ICU. N Engl J Med 2006; 355(26):2725–32.

[42] Lazar RM, Shapiro PA, Jaski BE, et al. Neurological events during long-term mechanical circulatory support for heart failure: the randomized evaluation of mechanical assistance for the treatment of congestive heart failure (REMATCH) experience. Circulation 2004;109:2423–7.

[43] Kalya AV, Tector AJ, Crouch JD, et al. Comparison of Novacor and HeartMate vented electric left ventricular assist devices in a single institution. J Heart Lung Transplant 2005;24:1973–5.

[44] Guthikonda S, Lev EI, Kleiman NS. Resistance to antiplatelet therapy. Curr Cardiol Rep 2005;7: 242–8.

[45] Rieder MJ, Reiner AP, Gage BF, et al. Effect of VKORC1 Haplotypes on transcriptional regulation and warfarin dose. N Engl J Med 2005;352: 2285–93.

[46] Flynn JD, Camp PC Jr, Jahania MS, et al. Successful treatment of refractory bleeding after bridging from acute to chronic left ventricular assist device support with recombinant activated factor VII. ASAIO J 2004;50(5):519–21.

[47] Frazier OH, Dowling RD, Gray LA Jr, et al. The total artificial heart: where we stand. Cardiology 2004;101:117–21.

[48] Kogan A, Berman M, Kassif Y, et al. Use of recombinant factor VII to control bleeding in a patient supported by right ventricular assist device after heart transplantation. J Heart Lung Transplant 2005;24(3):347–9.

[49] Potapov EV, Pasic M, Bauer M, et al. Activated recombinant factor VII for control of diffuse

bleeding after implantation of ventricular assist device. Ann Thorac Surg 2002;74(6):2182–3.

[50] Tual L, Kirsch M, Servant JM, et al. rFVIIa administration in patient with a left ventricular assistance patient. Ann Fr Anesth Reanim 2006;25(1): 29–32.

[51] Martin J, Siegenthaler MP, Friesewinkel O, et al. Implantable left ventricular assist device for treatment of pulmonary hypertension in candidates for orthotopic heart transplantation-a preliminary study. Eur J Cardiothorac Surg 2004;25:971–7.

[52] Salzberg SP, Lachat ML, von Harbou K, et al. Normalization of high pulmonary vascular resistance with LVAD support in heart transplantation candidates. Eur J Cardiothorac Surg 2005;27:222–5.

[53] Dang NC, Topkara VK, Mercando M, et al. Right heart failure after left ventricular assist device implantation in patients with chronic congestive heart failure. J Heart Lung Transplant 2006;25(1): 1–6.

[54] Oz MC, Goldstein DJ, Pepino P, et al. Screening scale predicts patients successfully receiving long-term implantable left ventricular assist devices. Circulation 1995;92(9 Suppl):II169–73.

[55] Rao V, Oz MC, Flannery MA, et al. Revised screening scale to predict survival after insertion of a left ventricular assist device. J Thorac Cardiovasc Surg 2003;125:855–62.

[56] Santambrogio L, Bianchi T, Fuardo M, et al. Right ventricular failure after left ventricular assist device insertion: preoperative risk factors. Interactive Cardiovascular and Thoracic Surgery 2006;5: 379–82.

[57] Field ME, Solomon SD, Lewis EF, et al. Right ventricular dysfunction and adverse outcome in patients with advanced heart failure. J Card Fail 2006;12(8):616–20.

[58] Fukamachi K, Horvath DJ, Massiello AL, et al. Development of a small implantable right ventricular assist device. ASAIO J 2005;51(6):730–5.

[59] Christiansen S, Perez-Bouza A, Reul H, et al. In vivo experimental testing of a microaxial blood pump for right ventricular support. Artif Organs 2006;30(2):94–100.

[60] Klodell CT Jr, Morey TE, Lobato EB, et al. Effect of sildenafil on pulmonary artery pressure, systemic pressure, and nitric oxide utilization in patients with left ventricular assist devices. Ann Thorac Surg 2007;83(1):68–71.

[61] Dowling RD, Park SJ, Pagani FD, et al. HeartMate VE LVAS design enhancements and its impact on device reliability. Eur J Cardiothorac Surg 2004;25:958–63.

[62] Dowling RD, Gray LA Jr, Etoch SW, et al. Initial experience with the AbioCor implantable replacement heart system. J Thorac Cardiovasc Surg 2004;127(1):131–41.

[63] Birks EJ, Tansley PD, Yacoub MH, et al. Incidence and clinical management of life-threatening left

ventricular assist device failure. J Heart Lung Transplant 2004;23:964–9.

[64] Pagani FD, Long JW, Dembitsky WP, et al. Improved mechanical reliability of the HeartMate XVE left ventricular assist system. Ann Thorac Surg 2006;82(4):1413–8.

[65] Martin J, Friesewinkel O, Benk C, et al. Improved durability of the HeartMate XVE left ventricular assist device provides safe mechanical support up to 1 year but is associated with high risk of device failure in the second year. J Heart Lung Transplant 2006;25(4):384–90.

[66] Mussivand T, Hetzer R, Vitali E, et al. Clinical results with an ePTFE inflow conduit for mechanical circulatory support. J Heart Lung Transplant 2004; 23(12):1366–70.

[67] Westaby S, Frazier OH, Banning A. Six years of continuous mechanical circulatory support. N Engl J Med 2006;355:325–7.

[68] Slaughter M. Destination therapy: the future is arriving. Congest Heart Fail 2005;11:155–6.

[69] Lietz K, Long J, Kfoury AG, et al. The impct of patient selection on long-term outcomes of left-ventricular assist device implantation as destination therapy for endstage heart failure (abstr). J Heart Lung Transplant 2006;25(2 Suppl):S131.

[70] Faggian G, Santini F, Franchi G, et al. Insights from continued use of a Novacor Left Ventricular Assist System for a period of 6 years. J Heart Lung Transplant 2005;24:1444.

[71] Feller ED, Sorensen EN, Haddad M, et al. Clinical outcomes are similar in pulsatile and nonpulsatile left ventricular assist device recipients. Ann Thorac Surg 2007;83(3):1082–8.

[72] Deng MC, Naka Y. Mechanical circulatory support therapy in advanced heart failure. London: Imperial College Press; 2007.

[73] Frazier OH, Kirklin JK. Mechanical circulatory support. ISHLT Monograph Series, Volume 1. Philadelphia: Elsevier; 2006.

[74] Baddour LM, Bettmann MA, Bolger AF, et al. Nonvalvular cardiovascular device-related infections. Clin Infect Dis 2004;38(8):1128–30.

[75] Schmid C, Tjan TD, Etz C, et al. First clinical experience with the Incor left ventricular assist device. J Heart Lung Transplant 2005;24:1188–94.

[76] Vitali E, Lanfranconi M, Ribera E, et al. Successful experience in bridging patients to heart transplantation with the MicroMed DeBakey ventricular assist device. Ann Thorac Surg 2003;75(4):1200–4.

[77] Gordon RJ, Quagliarello B, Lowy FD. Ventricular assist device-related infections. Lancet Infect Dis 2006;6(7):426–37.

[78] Klotz S, Stypmann J, Welp H, et al. Does continuous flow left ventricular assist device technology have a positive impact on outcome pretransplant and posttransplant? Ann Thorac Surg 2006;82: 1774–8.

[79] Fynn-Thompson F, Almond C. Pediatric Ventricular Assist Devices. Pediatr Cardiol 2007;28: 149–55.

[80] Minami K, El-Banayosy A, Sezai A, et al. Morbidity and outcome after mechanical ventricular support using Thoratec, Novacor, and HeartMate for bridging to heart transplantation. Artif Organs 2000;24:421–6.

[81] Schmid C, Debus V, Gogarten W, et al. Pediatric assist with the Medos and Excor systems in small children. ASAIO J 2006;52(5):505–8.

[82] Baldwin JT, Borovetz HS, Duncan BW, et al. The National Heart, Lung, and Blood Institute Pediatric Circulatory Support Program. Circulation 2006;113:147–55.

[83] Klotz S, Deng MC, Wilhelm MJ, et al. Left ventricular pressure and volume unloading during pulsatile versus non-pulsatile LVAD-support. Ann Thorac Surg 2004;77:143–9.

[84] Thohan V, Stetson SJ, Nagueh SF, et al. Cellular and hemodynamics responses of failing myocardium to continuous flow mechanical circulatory support using the DeBakey-Noon left ventricular assist device: a comparative analysis with pulsatile-type devices. J Heart Lung Transplant 2005; 24(5):566–75.

[85] Ündar A. Myths and truths of pulsatile and nonpulsatile perfusion during acute and chronic cardiac support. Artif Organs 2004;28(5):439–43.

[86] Bourque K, Dague C, Farrar D, et al. In vivo assessment of a rotary left ventricular assist device-induced artificial pulse in the proximal and distal aorta. Artif Organs 2006;30(8):638–42.

[87] Myers TJ, Palanichamy N, La Francesca S, et al. Management of multiple left ventricular assist device failures in a patient. J Heart Lung Transplant 2007;26(1):98–100.

[88] Ankersmit HJ, Tugulea S, Spanier T, et al. Activation-induced T-cell death and immune dysfunction after implantation of left-ventricular assist device. Lancet 1999;354(9178):550–5.

[89] Miller LW, Nelson KE, Bostic RR, et al. Hospital costs for left ventricular assist devices for destination therapy: lower costs for implantation in the post-REMATCH era. J Heart Lung Transplant 2006;25:778–84.

[90] Clegg AJ, Scott DA, Loveman E, et al. The clinical and cost-effectiveness of left ventricular assist devices for end-stage heart failure: a systematic review and economic evaluation. Health Technol Assess 2005;9(45):1–148.

[91] Digiorgi PL, Reel MS, Thornton B, et al. Heart transplant and left ventricular assist device costs. J Heart Lung Transplant 2005;24:200–4.

[92] Sharples LD, Dyer M, Cafferty F, et al. Cost-effectiveness of ventricular assist device use in the United Kingdom: results from the evaluation of ventricular assist device programme in the UK

(EVAD-UK). J Heart Lung Transplant 2006; 25(11):1336–43.

[93] Smetana GW, Lawrence VA, Cornell JE, et al. Preoperative pulmonary risk stratification for non-cardiothoracic surgery: systematic review for the American College of Physicians. Ann Intern Med 2006;144:581–95.

[94] Stevenson LW, Miller LW, Desvigne-Nickens P, et al. Left ventricular assist device as destination for patients undergoing intravenous inotropic therapy: a subset analysis from REMATCH (Randomized Evaluation of Mechanical Assistance in Treatment of Chronic Heart Failure). Circulation 2004;110:975–81.

[95] DeRose JJ Jr, Umana JP, Argenziano M, et al. Implantable left ventricular assist devices provide an excellent outpatient bridge to transplantation and recovery. J Am Coll Cardiol 1997;30(7):1773–7.

[96] McCarthy PM, Smedira NO, Vargo RL, et al. One hundred patients with the HeartMate left ventricular assist device: evolving concepts and technology. J Thorac Cardiovasc Surg 1998; 115(4):904–12.

[97] Schmid C, Hammel D, Deng MC, et al. Ambulatory care of patients with left ventricular assist devices. Circulation 1999;100(Suppl II):II-224–8.

[98] Weitkemper HH, El-Banayosy A, Arusoglu L, et al. Mechanical circulatory support: reality and dreams experience of a single center. J Extra Corpor Technol 2004;36:169–73.

[99] El-Banayosy A, Arusoglu L, Kizner L, et al. Novacor left ventricular assist system versus Heartmate vented electric left ventricular assist system as a long-term mechanical circulatory support device in bridging patients: a prospective study. J Thorac Cardiovasc Surg 2000;119:581–7.

[100] Asai T, Lee MH, Arrecubieta C, et al. Cellular coating of the left ventricular assist device textured polyurethane membrane reduces adhesion of Staphylococcus aureus. J Thorac Cardiovasc Surg 2007;113:1147–53.

[101] Hammel D, Tjan DT, Scheld HH, et al. Successful treatment of a Novacor LVAD malfunction without repeat sternotomy. Thorac Cardiovasc Surg 1998;46:154–6.

[102] Simsir SA, Lin SS, Ellis MF, et al. HeartMate XVE malfunction caused by fluid aspiration into the vent port. J Thorac Cardiovasc Surg 2004;128(4):619–21.

[103] Chinn R, Dembitsky W, Eaton L, et al. Multicenter experience: prevention and management of left ventricular assist device infections. ASAIO J 2005;51:461–70.

[104] Park SJ, Tector A, Piccioni W, et al. Left ventricular assist devices as destination therapy: a new look at survival. J Thorac Cardiovasc Surg 2005;129:9–17.

[105] Koul B, Solem JO, Steen S, et al. HeartMate left ventricular assist device as bridge to heart transplantation. Ann Thorac Surg 1998;65:1625–30.

[106] Korfer R, El-Banayosy A, Arusoglu L, et al. Single-center experience with the thoratec ventricular assist device. J Thorac Cardiovasc Surg 2000;119:596–600.

[107] Frazier OH, Rose EA, Oz MC, et al. HeartMate LVAS Investigators. Left Ventricular Assist System. Multicenter clinical evaluation of the HeartMate vented electric left ventricular assist system in patients awaiting heart transplantation. J Thorac Cardiovasc Surg 2001;122:1186–95.

[108] Dang NC, Topkara VK, Kim BT, et al. Clinical outcomes in patients with chronic congestive heart failure who undergo left ventricular assist device implantation. J Thorac Cardiovasc Surg 2005; 130:1302–9.

[109] Frazier O, Myers T, Palanichamy N, et al. Initial clinical experience with the Heartmate II left ventricular assist system. The Journal of Heart and Lung Transplantation 2006;25(2):149.

[110] Siegenthaler MP, Frazier OH, Beyersdorf F, et al. Mechanical reliability of the Jarvik 2000 Heart. Ann Thorac Surg 2006;81:1752–8.

[111] Leprince P, Bonnet N, Rama A, et al. Bridge to transplantation with the Jarvik-7 (CardioWest) total artificial heart: a single-center 15-year experience. J Heart Lung Transplant 2003;22:1296–303.

[112] Deng MC, Loebe M, El-Banayosy A, et al. Mechanical circulatory support for advanced heart failure: effect of patient selection on outcome. Circulation 2001;103:231–7.

[113] Portner PM, Jansen PG, Oyer PE, et al. Improved outcomes with an implantable left ventricular assist system: a multicenter study. Ann Thorac Surg 2001;71:205–9.

[114] Copeland JG, Smith RG, Arabia FA, et al. CardioWest Total Artificial Heart Investigators. Cardiac replacement with a total artificial heart as a bridge to transplantation. N Engl J Med 2004; 351:859–67.

[115] El Banayosy A, Arusoglu L, Morshuis M, et al. CardioWest total artificial heart: Bad Oeynhausen experience. Ann Thorac Surg 2005;80:548–52.

ELSEVIER
SAUNDERS

Heart Failure Clin 3 (2007) 369–375

Lifetime Circulatory Support Must Not Be Restricted to Transplant Centers

Stephen Westaby, MS, PhD, FRCS*

Oxford Heart Centre, John Radcliffe Hospital, Oxford, UK

The problem

Chronic heart failure affects around 5 million North Americans and 7 million Europeans each year, accounting for 2% of the total health care budget in Western countries [1]. The major component of health care costs is repeated hospital admissions to palliate intolerable symptoms and escalate medical treatment. It is estimated that between 250,000 and 500,000 patients in the United States and approximately 2.2 million worldwide are in the terminal phase of heart failure (Stage D, New York Heart Association [NYHA] IV) and refractory to maximum medical therapy [2]. With around 10% of the population older than 65 years of age suffering systolic left ventricular dysfunction, the number of patients who have heart failure will double within the next 25 years. In this global context cardiac transplantation is irrelevant. Essentially restricted to patients younger than 65 years of age who do not have significant comorbidity, fewer than 2,200 donor hearts per year are made available in the United States and around 150 in the United Kingdom [3]. In a population constantly bombarded with media coverage of medical advances, there will be escalating demand for relief from severely symptomatic Stage D disease. Provided with an effective treatment, most civilized health care systems are prepared to intervene irrespective of cost. The treatment of advanced renal disease sets the precedent. Hemodialysis, which provides an overall 60%

2-year survival in the United States, is offered irrespective of age or transplant eligibility at a cost of around $60,000 per year [4].

The strategy of lifetime left ventricular assist device (LVAD) deployment is based on the success of mechanical bridge to transplantation [5]. First-generation LVADs were designed to replace the failing left ventricle by providing stroke volume and pulsatile blood flow (Fig. 1a, b) [6]. Blood is actively withdrawn from the dilated chamber and pumped in a pulsatile manner to the ascending aorta at a rate of between 4 and 10 L/min. In patients dying of cardiogenic shock these devices sustain life until a donor organ is available, provide symptomatic relief, reverse multiorgan dysfunction, and attenuate the cytokine and humeral responses to heart failure [7]. Transplant outcomes are improved because terminally ill patients are in better condition to survive major surgery [8]. In turn comes the observation that mechanical unloading of the failing heart and increased coronary blood flow have important beneficial effects on the diseased myocardium. Reduced wall tension and stroke work result in decreased myocyte hypertrophy, apoptosis, myocytolysis, and fibrosis. Myocyte genetic expression and metabolic processes revert toward normal [9]. As a result LVADs can occasionally be removed following functional improvement of the native heart (Fig. 2) [10]. Bridge to recovery occurs more often in inflammatory conditions, such as myocarditis, intoxication, or idiopathic dilated cardiomyopathy.

With the exception of the United States, Germany, and France, bridge to transplantation is an expensive and infrequent intervention. In the study by Sharples and colleagues [11] evaluating the ventricular assist device program in the United

---
* Oxford Heart Centre, John Radcliffe Hospital, Headley Way, Headington, Oxford OX3 9DU, United Kingdom.

E-mail address: swestaby@AHF.org.uk

1551-7136/07/$ - see front matter © 2007 Elsevier Inc. All rights reserved.
doi:10.1016/j.hfc.2007.05.008

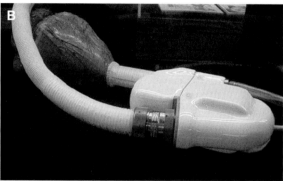

Fig. 1. (*A*) The HeartMate vented electric (VE) LVAD used in the REMATCH trial. (*Courtesy of* Thoratec Inc., Pleasanton, CA; with permission.) (*B*) The Novacor LVAD, which has sustained patients for more than 5 years.

Kingdom, only 70 LVADs were implanted in 32 months and 30 of these patients (43%) died before transplantation. Thirty-one (44%) completed bridge to transplantation, whereas 4 (6%) recovered without a transplant. Overall 12-month survival was 52%. Mean LVAD implant cost alone was around $120,000, although the pump was used only for weeks or months. In health care

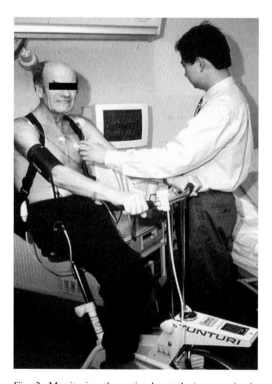

Fig. 2. Monitoring the native heart during exercise in a destination therapy patient with the HeartMate VE LVAD.

systems with limited resources LVADs might prove more cost effective for lifetime circulatory support in the non–transplant-eligible population.

Lifetime LVAD use (destination therapy) has a firm evidence base in the REMATCH trial (Randomized Evaluation of Mechanical Assistance for Treatment of Congestive Heart failure) [12]. This study was performed because of stringent limitations in transplant eligibility and because many LVAD patients were surviving for many months or years with good quality of life before a donor heart became available. Terminally ill NHYA Class IV non–transplant-eligible candidates were randomly assigned to a pulsatile first-generation LVAD or continued medical therapy. With an average age of 65 years, this population was older and sicker than conventional heart transplant candidates. At enrollment 68% required intravenous inotropes and the remainder had a peak myocardial oxygen consumption of 9.18 mL/kg/min, highly predictive of early mortality. Median survival in those assigned to the LVAD group was 409 days versus 150 days for controls managed medically. The 75% annual mortality for controls exceeded that for AIDS and many cancers. Although LVAD survival was disappointing, the device provided a 48% reduction in mortality during follow-up and a 27% reduction at 1 year.

It was soon clear that LVAD implant mortality was associated with established multiorgan failure, which proved refractory to an increase in systemic blood flow. The patient, not the device, was responsible for early attrition. With more reasonable patient selection, the initial modest 21% 2-year survival improved to 43% later in the trial. With a slightly modified blood pump, some centers now achieve 85% 1-year and 65% 2-year survival, which parallels that for hemodialysis in end-stage renal disease. There are other similarities between these end-stage populations. Chronic hemodialysis is only able to sustain life for several years in younger and otherwise healthy patients. When the number of patients older than 65 years of age increased to 80%, the overall 2-year survival for hemodialysis decreased to 60%. The average life expectancy for older hemodialysis patients is 2.6 years [13].

As experience increases, the strategic boundaries between bridge to transplantation, bridge to recovery, or lifetime use no longer exist. The LVAD sustains life, whereas the patient's response determines the clinical course. For instance, non–transplant-eligible patients may be salvaged with a temporary device and then switched to lifetime therapy should the heart not recover. If a transplant candidate's heart improves during LVAD unloading, there is the option for device removal instead of transplantation. In the future LVADs may also provide the platform for myocardial regeneration by neoangiogenesis, gene therapy, or stem cell therapy [14].

In REMATCH, late deaths occurred not through heart failure but from LVAD mechanical failure (35%), infective complications (41%), or stroke (10%). Advances in blood pump bioengineering have already dramatically reduced these risks [15]. Important developments include the fact that high-speed impellers do not damage red or white blood cells and that attenuated pulse pressure is well tolerated in the long term by the human circulation [16]. External components can be made exchangeable to combat wear and tear and the product is more user friendly for surgeon and patient (Fig. 3) [17].

In July 2006 the New England Journal of Medicine reported 6-year survival in the first patient to receive a miniaturized axial flow pump for lifetime use [18]. The Jarvik 2000 LVAD (Jarvik Heart, New York) was tested in laboratory programs in Houston and Oxford (Fig. 4a, b). The 61-year-old English patient had idiopathic dilated cardiomyopathy with longstanding biventricular failure. He was breathless at rest with pitting edema to the thighs, ulcerated legs, and ascites. Left ventricular ejection fraction was less than 10%. He was rejected for cardiac transplantation because of renal impairment and subsequently declined the procedure. Almost 7 years later he is NYHA Class II with an active life in the community. Pump output is around 5.0

L/min against a mean blood pressure of between 70 to 80 mm Hg, usually with a pulse pressure of 10 to 15 mm Hg. Power is delivered by way of a skull-mounted titanium pedestal, which has remained infection free (see Fig. 3). The external cables, controller, and batteries have all required exchange for wear and tear. Less than 5% of the follow-up period has been spent in hospital and total cost has been around $200,000.

After extensive laboratory testing suggested that continuous pump flow and attenuated pulse pressure were safe in the long term, the Oxford Group proceeded to a pilot study of lifetime support in nine Stage D patients who had end-stage dilated cardiomyopathy. All had been turned down for cardiac transplantation because of renal dysfunction with or without elevated pulmonary vascular resistance. Two died in hospital from right heart and multiorgan failure. Three are alive and well without an adverse event between 13 months and 6.8 years postoperatively. Three others have died at 12 months, 26 months, 35 months postoperatively, all from noncardiac causes. A fourth patient had enjoyed 3.5 years of event-free independent life more than 200 miles away from the implanting center. He died of acute left ventricular failure after failing to take a replacement battery on an excursion. At autopsy in all these patients the pump and vascular graft were free from thrombosis and there were no signs of thromboembolism. The skull pedestal remained free from infection in each case. The explanted LVADs continued to function normally on the bench. So far the Jarvik 2000 has proven to be 100% mechanically reliable in 150 implants and has a lower complication rate than pulsatile pumps [19].

Careful medical management plays an important part in the symbiotic relationship between a rotary blood pump and an improving native heart. These LVADs are particularly sensitive to differential pressure across the rotor (afterload) [15]. An increase in peripheral vascular resistance can dramatically reduce pump flow leading to renewed symptoms. The patients benefit from continuous afterload reduction by angiotensin-converting enzyme inhibition, a beta-blocker, or both. The native heart responds to exercise by increasing cardiac output through the apical LVAD and the aortic valve. Longstanding Jarvik 2000 patients are maintained with a mean systemic blood pressure of 60 to 70 mm Hg and little more than 10 to 20 mm Hg pulse pressure [18]. They can exercise without changing the pump speed from 10,000 rpm.

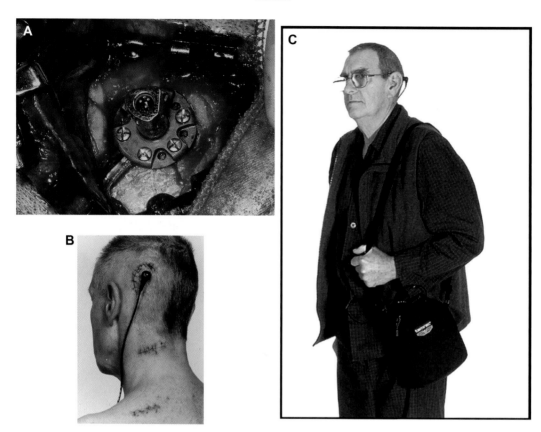

Fig. 3. Skull pedestal technique for completely exchangeable components of the Jarvik Flowmaker LVAD: (*A*) Titanium pedestal screwed to the skull. (*Courtesy of* Oxford Medical Illustration, Oxford, UK; with permission.) (*B*) The power line attached to the pedestal. (*C*) Easily portable external components: controller and battery. (*Courtesy of* Oxford Medical Illustration, Oxford, UK; with permission.)

This preliminary lifetime support experience with rotary blood pumps suggests the need for another REMATCH-type study, this time targeting patients who have debilitating symptoms (NYHA III/IV) that restrict independent life in the community. As an end point, quality of life should assume equal importance to survival. A control group is justified because the patient cohort is sufficiently different from REMATCH (less sick).

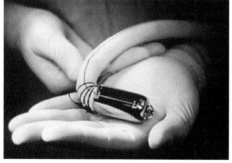
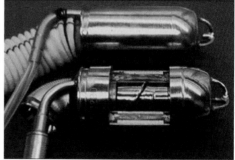

Fig. 4. The "thumb-sized" Jarvik Flowmaker pump, which is implanted into the apex of the failing left ventricle.

How to increase the delivery of long term circulatory support

There are around 60,000 Stage D heart failure patients younger than 65 years in the United States and 12,000 in the United Kingdom [2]. Given the availability of LVADs with mechanical reliability beyond 5 years, is it morally justified to withhold an "off the shelf" solution for a proportion of these patients? The Health Care Advisory Board (USA) has predicted that mechanical circulatory support will be the principal treatment option for advanced heart failure by the year 2010. More than 100,000 devices are expected to be implanted annually in the United States at a cost of around $11 billion. This development requires a change in current philosophy.

Rotary blood pumps are not yet available for lifetime circulatory support in the United States (Fig. 5a–d). Although outcomes with the Heart-Mate (Thoratec Corporation, Pleasanton, California) and Novacor (World Heart Corporation, Ottawa, Ontario, Canada) LVADs have progressively improved, their size, complexity, and complication rates have constrained more widespread use in the community. In contrast the user-friendly rotary blood pumps could be used at an earlier stage of the disease process for symptomatic relief and attenuation of the remodeling process.

In the future, LVADs will be implantable without major thoracic surgery or cardiopulmonary bypass. Blood pumps will then be used alongside cardiac resynchronization therapy and implantable defibrillators in all major cardiac centers. Now that mainstream surgical centers are equipped with short-term circulatory support devices for postcardiotomy or postangioplasty salvage, long-term support with an implantable LVAD is a relatively small step. With rotary blood pumps the operation is usually simple and the postoperative care is completely different from transplantation. Lifetime LVAD use must be undertaken electively for symptomatic relief and not as a salvage procedure for multisystem organ failure. The elective approach greatly simplifies the perioperative management of this high-risk non–transplant-eligible population.

Recruitment of centers to perform lifetime circulatory support

After the REMATCH trial the International Society for Heart and Lung Transplantation (ISHLT) assembled a committee of heart failure cardiologists and transplant surgeons to define the minimum requirements for long-term circulatory support centers. At the time the HeartMate pulsatile LVAD was the only product licensed for chronic therapy in the United States and the options were limited as follows:

Option 1: Restrict long-term LVAD implantation to REMATCH participating heart transplant centers.

Option 2: Restrict long-term LVAD implantation to heart transplant centers currently experienced with bridge to transplantation, assuming that only these centers can provide expertise to perform at levels that ensure outcomes comparable to REMATCH.

Option 3: Use a staged approach. For Stage 1 restrict long term LVAD programs to hospitals as defined in Option 2. For Stage 2 expand to nontransplant centers with established long-term cooperation with a regional cardiac transplant program as long as these centers meet a minimum set of requirements for training and infrastructure. This option acknowledged that demand could outstrip the capacity of transplant centers to perform and care for long-term patients.

Option 4: Allow long-term LVAD programs in all interested hospitals with cardiac surgery programs but continuously monitor center-specific outcomes with further approval based on achieving a target outcome. The rationale for this option is that all centers that perform cardiac surgery should have equal opportunity to use devices for non–transplant-eligible patients according to the same procedural algorithms.

Option 5: Define a minimum set of requirements for training of physicians, surgeons, and other personnel and infrastructure, before initiating long-term LVAD programs in all interested centers. Use assessment of center-specific outcomes on an annual basis with continued approval based on achieving target outcomes. This approach balances safety issues with the priority to disseminate LVAD therapy for the benefit of the large advanced heart failure population without access to heart transplantation.

Option 5 was the preferred strategy of the ISHLT Board of Directors. The ISHLT recommends that each center should have an established heart failure program directed by specialized heart failure cardiologists who have experience in end-stage disease. Some cardiologists and cardiac

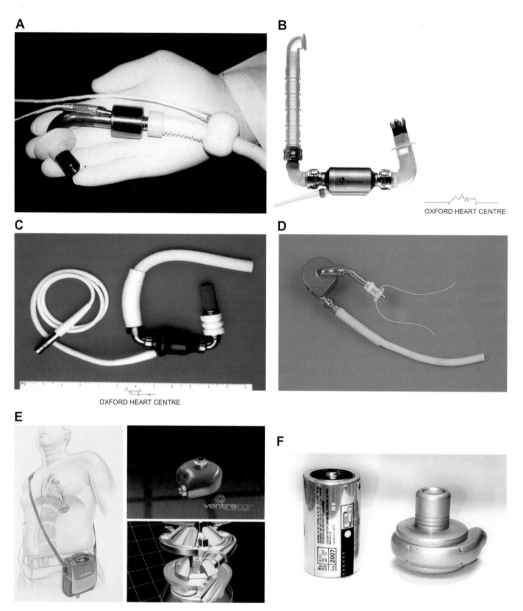

Fig. 5. Rotary blood pumps now in clinical use: (*A*) Micromed DeBakey (Micromed Technology, Inc., Houston, Texas). (*B*) Berline Incor (Berlin Heart, Berlin, Germany). (*C*) Thermo Cardio Systems II (Thoractec Corporation, Pleasanton, California). (*D*) Terumo Duraheart (Terumo, Inc., Japan). (*E*) Ventracor (Ventracor, Australia). (*F*) Heartware (Florida) LVAD next to a "D" cell battery.

surgeons should have worked in a cardiac transplant center and with the management of bridge-to-transplant patients. At least one surgeon must have documented expertise in LVAD implantation, perioperative and postoperative management, and removal of such devices. Other participating physicians and surgeons should have adequate training through educational fellowships or programs conducted at an established LVAD center. Also recommended is a comprehensive infrastructure for noncardiac medical and surgical issues, infectious disease management, LVAD nursing, and social work. Written protocols should be provided for pre-, intra-, and postoperative LVAD management, including end-of-life situations. The center should have quality assurance programs and include participation in the ISHLT LVAD database. Highly desirable is an advanced heart failure research and teaching program to support patient care.

Oxford, a nontransplant center with an interest in conventional heart failure surgery, began an LVAD laboratory research program in 1995. This program provided substantial experience in LVAD implantation and postoperative care with several short- and long-term devices that have now transferred to the clinical arena. This experience was the basis on which to build a successful program with the experience of maintaining LVAD patients in the community for more than 7 years and bridge-to-recovery survival exceeding 9 years. This program is an ISHLT option 5 and a model on which to develop nontransplant heart failure centers. The manufacturers of circulatory support systems now aim to provide technology that is simple and safe to use in centers that do not have the infrastructure required for cardiac transplantation.

Heart failure that does not respond to maximum medical management is a frightening and debilitating condition. The patients have poor quality of life and become progressively more dependent on hospital admissions for escalating medical therapy. Long-term circulatory support can provide symptomatic relief and improved survival for those who do not have access to cardiac transplantation. User-friendly blood pumps with proven durability already exist. In a society that provides renal support for patients irrespective of age, is it justified to withhold circulatory support when this seems to be cost effective by reducing the frequency of hospital admissions? To provide this service, rotary blood pumps must be made available in centers other than those involved in transplantation. The mystique should be removed from this relatively simple intervention.

References

[1] Stewart S. Financial aspects of heart failure programs of care. Eur J Heart Fail 2005;7:423–8.

[2] Redfield MM. Heart failure—an epidemic of uncertain proportions. N Engl J Med 2002;347:1442–4.

[3] Hunt SA. Taking heart—cardiac transplantation, past, present and future. N Engl J Med 2006;355:231–5.

[4] Lee H, Mans B, Taub K, et al. Cost analysis of ongoing care of patients with end stage renal disease: the impact of dialysis modality and dialysis access. Am J Kidney Dis 2002;40:611–22.

[5] Navia JL, McCarthy PM, Hoercher KJ, et al. Do left ventricular assist device (LVAD) bridge to transplant outcomes predict the results of permanent LVAD implantation. Ann Thorac Surg 2002;74:2051–63.

[6] Kayala AV, Tector AJ, Crouch JD, et al. Comparison of Novacor and HeartMate vented electric left ventricular assist devices in a single institution. J Heart Lung Transplant 2005;11:1973–5.

[7] Pae WE, Miller CA, Mathews Y, et al. Ventricular assist devices for postcardiotomy cardiogenic shock. A combined registry experience. J Thorac Cardiovasc Surg 1992;104:541–53.

[8] Frazier OH, Rose AN, McCarthy PM, et al. Improved mortality and rehabilitation of transplant candidates treated with a long-term implantable left ventricular assist device. Ann Surg 1995;222:327–8.

[9] Zhang J, Narula J. Molecular biology of myocardial recovery. Surg Clin North Am 2004;84:223–42.

[10] Hetzer R, Muller J, Weng Y, et al. Cardiac recovery in dilated cardiomyopathy by unloading with a left ventricular assist device. Ann Thorac Surg 1999;68:742–9.

[11] Sharples LD, Buxton MJ, Caine N. Evaluation of the left ventricular assist device programme in the United Kingdom. J Heart Lung Transplant 2006;25(Suppl 1):80–1.

[12] Rose EA, Gelijns AC, Moskowitz AJ, et al. Randomised Evauation of Mechnical Assistance for the Treatment of Congestive Heart Failure (RE-MATCH) Study Group. Long-term mechanical left ventricular assistance for end-stage heart failure. N Engl J Med 2001;345:1435–43.

[13] The United States Renal Data System. 2004 annual data report. Available at: http://www.usrds.org/. Accessed June 15, 2007.

[14] Woller KC, Drexler H. Clinical applications of stem cells for the heart. Circ Res 2005;96:151–63.

[15] Westaby S. Ventricular assist device as destination therapy. Surg Clin North Am 2004;84:91–123.

[16] Saito S, Nishinaka T, Westaby S. Hemodynamics of chronic non-pulsatile flow: implications for development. Surg Clin North Am 2004;84:61–74.

[17] Westaby S, Jarvik R, Freeland A, et al. Post auricular percutaneous power delivery for permanent mechanical circulatory support. J Thorac Cardiovasc Surg 2002;123:977–83.

[18] Westaby S, Frazier OH, Banning A. Six years of continuous circulatory support. N Engl J Med 2006;355:325–7.

[19] Siegenthaler M, Frazier OH, Westaby S, et al. Mechanical reliability of the Jarvik 2000 Heart. Ann Thorac Surg 2006;81:1752–8.

ELSEVIER
SAUNDERS

Heart Failure Clin 3 (2007) 377–380

HEART
FAILURE
CLINICS

Index

Note: Page numbers of article titles are in **boldface** type.

A

Aldosterone antagonists, in advanced heart failure, 323

American Heart Association (AHA)/American College of Cardiology (ACC), management of heart failure and, 325

Angiotensin receptor blockers, in advanced heat failure, 324

Aortic regurgitation, chronic volume overload in, 293
conditions causing, 292–294
decision for aortic valve surgery in, 293
impaired systolic function in, 293
natural history of, 292–293
pressure overload in, 292
severe chronic, 293

Aortic stenosis, aortic valve replacement in, 294–295
causes of, 294
mild, natural history of, 294
transition from asymptomatic to symptomatic stage of, 294

Aortic valve, percutaneous replacement of, 296–297

Aortic valve disease, surgical treatment of, 292–295
tricuspid valve disease in, 295

Aortic valve replacement, in aortic stenosis, 294–295
return of congestive heart failure following, 295

Aortic valve surgery, decision for, in aortic regurgitation, 293
in advanced heart failure, 329–330

B

Biomedical devices, for heart failure, 295–296

C

Cardiac assist devices, mechanical, 299, 300

Cardiac defibrillator, automatic implantable, in advanced heart failure, 326–327
inflatable, 269

Cardiac resynchronization therapy. See *Resynchronization therapy.*

Cardiac support systems, fully implantable pulsatile, 299, 300

Cardiac transplantation. See *Transplantation, cardiac.*

Cardiomyopathy, dilated. See *Dilated cardiomyopathy.*
hypertrophic. See *Hypertrophic cardiomyopathy.*

Circulatory support, lifetime, must not be restricted to transplant centers, **369–375**
mechanical, in advanced heart failure, 331, 332

Coagulopathies, destination mechanical circulatory support devices and, 331, 353

Congestive heart failure. See *Heart failure, congestive.*

Coronary artery bypass surgery, in advanced heart failure, 328

Coronary interventions, percutaneous, in advanced heart failure, 327–328

D

Defibrillator, cardiac, automatic implantable, in advanced heart failure, 326–327
inflatable, 269

Destination mechanical circulatory support devices, adverse events associated with, incidence of, 352
areas of research for, 358
biocompatibility of, 362–363
clinical implementation delay and, 357
clinically evaluated, characteristics of, 354–355

Moving?

Make sure your subscription moves with you!

To notify us of your new address, find your **Clinics Account Number** (located on your mailing label above your name), and contact customer service at:

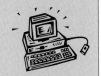

E-mail: elspcs@elsevier.com

800-654-2452 (subscribers in the U.S. & Canada)
407-345-4000 (subscribers outside of the U.S. & Canada)

Fax number: 407-363-9661

Elsevier Periodicals Customer Service
6277 Sea Harbor Drive
Orlando, FL 32887-4800

*To ensure uninterrupted delivery of your subscription, please notify us at least 4 weeks in advance of move.